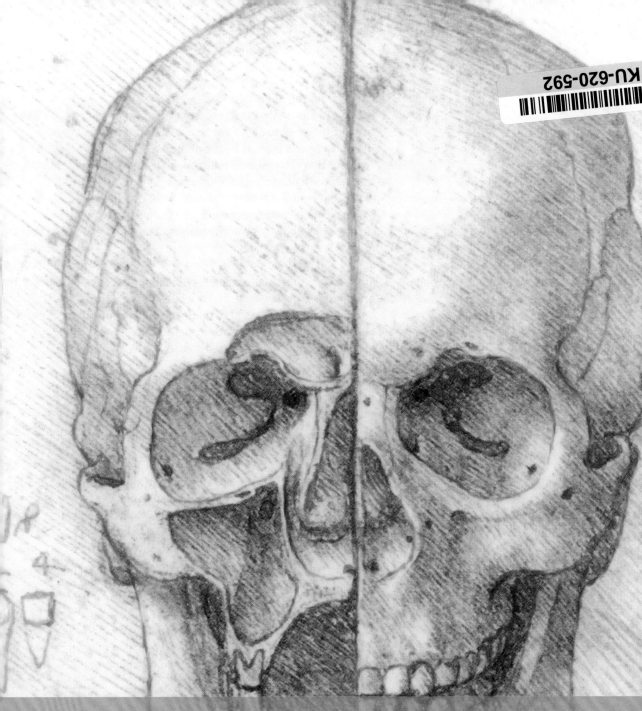

Edexcel GCSE (9-1)
History

WITHDRAWN

Medicine through time, c1250–present

Series Editor: Angela Leonard   Authors: Sally Thorne   Hilary Stark

PEARSON

Published by Pearson Education Limited, 80 Strand, London, WC2R 0RL.

www.pearsonschoolsandfecolleges.co.uk

Copies of official specifications for all Edexcel qualifications may be found on the website: www.edexcel.com

Text © Pearson Education Limited 2016

Series editor: Angela Leonard
Designed by Colin Tilley Loughrey, Pearson Education Limited
Typeset by Phoenix Photosetting, Chatham, Kent
Original illustrations © Pearson Education Limited
Illustrated by KJA Artists Illustration Agency and Phoenix Photosetting, Chatham, Kent.

Cover design by Colin Tilley Loughrey
Picture research by Christine Martin
Cover photo © Science Photo Library / Sheila Terry

The right of Hilary Stark and Sally Thorne to be identified as author of this work has been asserted by her in accordance with the Copyright, Designs and Patents Act 1988.

First published 2016

19 18 17
10 9 8 7 6 5 4

British Library Cataloguing in Publication Data
A catalogue record for this book is available from the British Library.
ISBN 978 1 292 12737 8

Printed in Slovakia by Neografia

A note from the publisher

In order to ensure that this resource offers high-quality support for the associated Pearson qualification, it has been through a review process by the awarding body. This process confirms that this resource fully covers the teaching and learning content of the specification or part of a specification at which it is aimed. It also confirms that it demonstrates an appropriate balance between the development of subject skills, knowledge and understanding, in addition to preparation for assessment.

Endorsement does not cover any guidance on assessment activities or processes (e.g. practice questions or advice on how to answer assessment questions), included in the resource nor does it prescribe any particular approach to the teaching or delivery of a related course.

While the publishers have made every attempt to ensure that advice on the qualification and its assessment is accurate, the official specification and associated assessment guidance materials are the only authoritative source of information and should always be referred to for definitive guidance.

Pearson examiners have not contributed to any sections in this resource relevant to examination papers for which they have responsibility.

Examiners will not use endorsed resources as a source of material for any assessment set by Pearson.

Endorsement of a resource does not mean that the resource is required to achieve this Pearson qualification, nor does it mean that it is the only suitable material available to support the qualification, and any resource lists produced by the awarding body shall include this and other appropriate resources.

Websites

Pearson Education Limited is not responsible for the content of any external internet sites. It is essential for tutors to preview each website before using it in class so as to ensure that the URL is still accurate, relevant and appropriate. We suggest that tutors bookmark useful websites and consider enabling students to access them through the school/college intranet.

Acknowledgements

Acknowledgements

Picture Credits
The publisher would like to thank the following for their kind permission to reproduce their photographs:

(Key: b-bottom; c-centre; l-left; r-right; t-top)

Alamy Images: Bruce McGowan 118l, Chronicle 160b, Everett Collection Historical 147l, GL Archive 77, 147r, GL Archive 77, 147r, Lebrecht Music and Arts Photo Library 155, 156, Lebrecht Music and Arts Photo Library 155, 156, Lordprice Collection 63, PRISMA ARCHIVO 28, Universal Images Group North America LLC 149l; **Bridgeman Art Library Ltd:** A map from 'On the Mode of Communication of Cholera', 1855 (litho), Snow, John (1813–58) (after) / Private Collection / Photo © Christie's Images 93, Anatomical Study, illustration from 'De Humani Corporis Fabrica' by Andreas Vesalius (1514–64) Basel, 1543 (engraving) (b / w photo), Vesalius, Andreas (1514–64) (after) / Bibliotheque des Arts Decoratifs, Paris, France / Archives Charmet 53r, Lansdowne 451 fol.127 A Leper with a Bell, from a Pontifical, c.1400 (vellum), English School, (15th century) / British Library, London, UK / © British Library Board. All Rights Reserved 10b, 14, Patients and nuns at the Hospital of Hotel Dieu in Paris, from 'Le Livre de Vie Active de l'Hotel Dieu' by Jean Henry, c.1482 (vellum), French School, (15th century) / Musee de l'Assistance Publique, Hopitaux de Paris, France / Archives Charmet 10t, 30, The Black Death, 1348 (engraving) (b&w photo), English School, (14th century) / Private Collection 32, Thomas Sydenham (1624–1689 A.D.) / Universal History Archive / UIG 44, Vein or Blood-letting Man / British Library, London, UK / © British Library Board. All Rights Reserved 24, War wounded arriving at a London train terminus, 1914–19 (litho), English School, (20th century) / Private Collection / The Stapleton Collection 136–137; **Frederick Sadler Brereton:** The great war and the R.A.M.C 158; **Getty Images:** BSIP 103, De Agostini Picture Library 13, DEA / A. DAGLI ORT 40, Hulton Archive 72, Italian School 19, Keystone 114, Paul Popper / Popperfoto 151, Peter Purdy 100, 118r, Popperfoto 162, Print Collector 56, Science & Society Picture Library 55, 171, Universal History Archive 68, 86, UniversalImagesGroup 91, 92; **Imperial War Museum:** 140, 157, 160t, © Crown Copyright 172; **Public Health England:** 115; **Radiography and radio-therapeutics Robert Knox:** 168, 178; **Science Photo Library Ltd:** 82, 102, OTIS HISTORICAL ARCHIVES, NATIONAL MUSEUM OF HEALTH AND MEDICINE 143; **The Royal Society:** 46; TopFoto: Topham Picture Point 113; **Wellcome Library, London:** 50; Wellcome Library, London: 53l, 58, 78, 79, 81, 94l, 94r

Cover images: *Front:* **Science Photo Library Ltd:** *Sheila Terry*

All other images © Pearson Education

Every effort has been made to trace the copyright holders and we apologise in advance for any unintentional omissions. We would be pleased to insert the appropriate acknowledgement in any subsequent edition of this publication.

We are grateful to the following for permission to reproduce copyright material:

Text
Extract in Source A on page 23 from *Medicine and society in late Medieval England*, New edition, (Rawcliffe,C. 1995) p.64, Sutton Publishing Ltd with permission; Extract in Interpretation 1 on page 35 from *A Short History of Disease*, Pocket Essentials (Martin,S. 2015) p.109 with permission from Oldcastle Books; Extract in Interpretation 1 on page 57, Harkness, Deborah E. "A View from the Streets: Women and Medical Work in Elizabethan London." Bulletin of the History of Medicine 82.1 (2008), 52–85. © 2008 The Johns Hopkins University Press. Reprinted with permission of Johns Hopkins University Press; Arnold, M.) 2012 Cambridge Scholars Publishing; Extract in Interpretation 1 on page 73 from *Disease Class and Social Change*, Cambridge Scholars Publishing (Arnold, M 2012) p.22; Extract in Source C on page 103 from Angelina Jolie undergoes double mastectomy after learning she had high risk of breast cancer, *The Mirror*, 14/05/2013 (Robertson, J); Extract in Source A on page 108 from Too much of a good thing (Shute J), © Copyright of Telegraph Media Group Limited 2013; Extract in Interpretation 1 on page 111 from *Health and Medicine in Britain since 1860 (Social History in Perspective*, Palgrave Macmillan (Anne Hardy) p.147, reproduced with permission of Palgrave Macmillan; Extract in Interpretation 2 on page 111 from The new NHS. modern. dependable, Presented to Parliament by the Secretary of State for Health by Command of Her Majesty, December 1997 Cm 3807 published by The Stationery Office as ISBN 0 10 138072 0, Contains public sector information licensed under the Open Government Licence v3.0; Extract in Source C on page 118 from Sir Alexander Fleming's speech at the Nobel Banquet, From Les Prix Nobel en 1945, Editor Arne Holmberg, [Nobel Foundation], Stockholm, 1946 Copyright © The Nobel Foundation 1945; Extract on page 119 from The Role Science Plays in Science Education, by (Harding,P.A.) p.134,© Copyright by Patricia Alice Harding, 1996; Extract in Source A on page 125 from Tobacco displays in shops to end from today Anne Milton MP 06/04/2012, Contains public sector information licensed under the Open Government Licence v3.0; Poetry in Source D on page 150 from *War Poems of Siegfried Sassoon*, Dover Publications (Siegfried, S.) p.59, copyright Siegfried Sassoon by kind permission of the Estate of George Sassoon; Extract in Source E on page 150 from *Diaries of a stretcher bearer 1916–18*, Boolarong Press (Edward, C.M., edited Munro,D. 2010) p.36; Extract in Source G on page 151 from Consolidated Fund (No. 3) BILL. HC Deb 23 June 1915 vol 72 cc1276-303, Sir J. D. REES, Contains Parliamentary information licensed under the Open Parliament Licence v3.0; Extract in Source A on page 154 from *Forgotten Voices of the Great War / IWM*, Ebury Press (Arthur, M / IWM 2002) p.100; Extract in Source C on page 155 from Fatal airs : the deadly history and apocalyptic future of lethal gases that threaten our world by Christianson, Scott Reproduced with permission of Praeger in the format Republish in a book via Copyright Clearance Center; Extract in Source F on page 156 from *The Gates of Memory*, OUP (Keynes, G 1981) p.129–130. By permission of Oxford University Press; Extract in Source C on page 159 from Private Papers of Major E S B Hamilton MC RAMC, © IWM 2016, with permission from The Trustees the Estate of Major ESB Hamilton MC RAMC; Extract in Source I on page 162 from *Forgotten Voices of the Great War*, Ebury Press (Arthur, M/ IWM); Extract in Source L page 164 from The Telegraph 1915, © Copyright of Telegraph Media Group Limited.

Contents

What's covered?

This book covers the Thematic study on Medicine through time and the Historical Environment, c1250 to present. These units make up 30% of your GCSE course, and will be examined in Paper 1.

Thematic studies cover a long period of history, and require you to know about change and continuity across different ages and aspects of society. You will need to know about key people, events and developments and make comparisons between the different periods studied.

Linked to the thematic study is a historic environment that examines a specific site and its relationship to historical events and developments.

Features

As well as a clear, detailed explanation of the key knowledge you will need, you will also find a number of features in the book:

Key terms

Where you see a word followed by an asterisk, like this: Salient*, you will be able to find a Key Terms box on that page that explains what the word means.

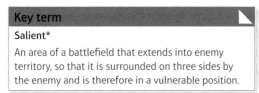

Key term

Salient*

An area of a battlefield that extends into enemy territory, so that it is surrounded on three sides by the enemy and is therefore in a vulnerable position.

Activities

Every few pages, you'll find a box containing some activities designed to help check and embed knowledge and get you to really think about what you've studied. The activities start simple, but might get more challenging as you work through them.

Summaries and Checkpoints

At the end of each chunk of learning, the main points are summarised in a series of bullet points – great for embedding the core knowledge, and handy for revision.

Checkpoints help you to check and reflect on your learning. The Strengthen section helps you to consolidate knowledge and understanding, and check that you've grasped the basic ideas and skills.

The Challenge questions push you to go beyond just understanding the information, and into evaluation and analysis of what you've studied.

Sources and Interpretations

This book contains numerous contemporary pictorial and text sources that show what people from the period, said, thought or created. You will need to be comfortable examining sources to answer questions in your Paper 1 exam.

Although interpretations do not appear in Paper 1, the book also includes extracts from the work of historians, showing how experts have interpreted the events you've been studying.

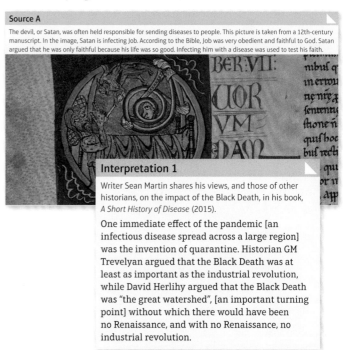

Source A

The devil, or Satan, was often held responsible for sending diseases to people. This picture is taken from a 12th-century manuscript. In the image, Satan is infecting Job. According to the Bible, Job was very obedient and faithful to God. Satan argued that he was only faithful because his life was so good. Infecting him with a disease was used to test his faith.

Interpretation 1

Writer Sean Martin shares his views, and those of other historians, on the impact of the Black Death, in his book, *A Short History of Disease* (2015).

One immediate effect of the pandemic [an infectious disease spread across a large region] was the invention of quarantine. Historian GM Trevelyan argued that the Black Death was at least as important as the industrial revolution, while David Herlihy argued that the Black Death was "the great watershed", [an important turning point] without which there would have been no Renaissance, and with no Renaissance, no industrial revolution.

Extend your knowledge

These features contain useful additional information that adds depth to your knowledge, and to your answers. The information is closely related to the key issues in the unit, and questions are sometimes included, helping you to link the new details to the main content.

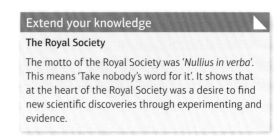

Extend your knowledge

The Royal Society

The motto of the Royal Society was 'Nullius in verba'. This means 'Take nobody's word for it'. It shows that at the heart of the Royal Society was a desire to find new scientific discoveries through experimenting and evidence.

Exam-style questions and tips

The book also includes extra exam-style questions you can use to practise. These appear in the chapters and are accompanied by a tip to help you get started on an answer.

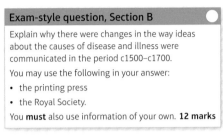

Exam-style question, Section B

Explain why there were changes in the way ideas about the causes of disease and illness were communicated in the period c1500–c1700.

You may use the following in your answer:

- the printing press
- the Royal Society.

You **must** also use information of your own. **12 marks**

Exam tip

Make sure that you fully explain your points by using the **P**oint, **E**xample, **E**xplain, or **PEE** method. State your argument, then add some examples from your own knowledge to back it up. Finish off by explaining how that evidence relates to the question.

Recap pages

At the end of each chapter, you'll find a page designed to help you to consolidate and reflect on the chapter as a whole. Each recap page includes a recall quiz, ideal for quickly checking your knowledge or for revision. Recap pages also include activities designed to help you summarise and analyse what you've learned, and also reflect on how each chapter links to other parts of the unit.

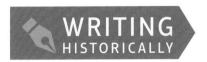

THINKING HISTORICALLY

These activities are designed to help you develop a better understanding of how history is constructed, and are focused on the key areas of Evidence, Interpretations, Cause & Consequence and Change & Continuity. In the Thematic Study, you will come across activities on both Cause and Change, and in the Historical Environment on Evidence, as these are key areas of focus for these units.

The Thinking Historically approach has been developed in conjunction with Dr Arthur Chapman and the Institute of Education, UCL. It is based on research into the misconceptions that can hold students back in history.

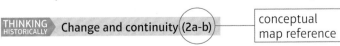

THINKING HISTORICALLY — Change and continuity (2a-b) — conceptual map reference

The Thinking Historically conceptual map can be found at: www.pearsonschools.co.uk/thinkinghistoricallygcse

WRITING HISTORICALLY

At the end of most chapters is a spread dedicated to helping you improve your writing skills. These include simple techniques you can use in your writing to make your answers clearer, more precise and better focused on the question you're answering.

The Writing Historically approach is based on the *Grammar for Writing* pedagogy developed by a team at the University of Exeter and popular in many English departments. Each spread uses examples from the preceding chapter, so it's relevant to what you've just been studying.

Preparing for your exams

At the back of the book, you'll find a special section dedicated to explaining and exemplifying the new Edexcel GCSE History exams. Advice on the demands of this paper, written by Angela Leonard, helps you prepare for and approach the exam with confidence. Each question type is explained through annotated sample answers at two levels, showing clearly how answers can be improved.

Pearson Progression Scale: This icon indicates the Step that a sample answer has been graded at on the Pearson Progression Scale.

This book is also available as an online ActiveBook, which can be licensed for your whole institution.

There is also an ActiveLearn Digital Service available to support delivery of this book, featuring a front-of-class version of the book, lesson plans, worksheets, exam practice PowerPoints, assessments, notes on Thinking Historically and Writing Historically, and more.

ActiveLearn
Digital Service

About change

This course is about two things: it is about the history of medicine, and it is about **change**. You are going to look at a long period of time – over 750 years. Medicine is the theme you will follow through these years. Concentrating on just one part of British life means you can also focus on how and why things change (and sometimes how and why they don't.)

This introduction is to help you understand the language and concepts historians use when they discuss change.

- **Change** – this is when things become different than they were before.
- **Continuity** – this is the opposite of change, when things stay the same, sometimes for a very long time.
- Change isn't always the same as **progress** – which is when things get better.
- The **rate of change** – change doesn't always happen at the same pace – sometimes things change very quickly, but sometimes they change slowly. Historians are interested in why this is.
- A **trend** is when there are a number of similar and related changes, continuing in the same direction, over a period of time – for example, the fact that there were 35 million people with smartphones in the UK in 2014 is part of the trend in the growing use of mobile phones.

- A **turning point** is when a significant change happens – something that is different from what has happened before and which will affect the future. For example, it was a turning point when Michael Harrison made the first ever mobile phone call in Britain on 1 January 1985.
- Historians are very interested in the **factors** that affect change. Some of them can be quite obvious, but others are more surprising. For example:
  - ♣ developments in science and technology, particularly around miniaturisation, have affected the development of the mobile phone
  - ♣ people's attitudes have also affected the development of the mobile phone. For example, text messaging (SMS) was not originally designed to be used – it was built in to help scientists test the first networks and phones. But users found out about it, liked it, and it has now become part of our world
  - ♣ less surprisingly, government has affected the development of mobile phones – with regulations about networks, laws about using them, and planning control of phone masts.

Look out for plenty more factors that affect change throughout the course.

Activities ?

1   Write your own definitions for each of the words in bold above, and explain your own example of each one.

2   Graphs can be a useful way to show change. Study the graph opposite.

   a   Where would you put these two factors affecting change on the graph? i) Worries about the health effects of butter are common. ii) Government campaigns to get people to reduce the fat in their diet.

   b   At the same time, bread sales fell by about 50%. Is this a factor affecting spread sales?

3   Study the table summarising Katy and Mel's journeys to school.

   a   Draw a line graph, with two lines, showing Katy and Mel's independence in their journeys. On the x-axis have the school years from 1 to 11. On the y-axis, plot their independence. For each of them, score their two journeys (to and from

school) and add the scores together. Going with a parent: scores 1 mark; using public transport: 2 marks; going by themselves: 3 marks. (Use half marks when they sometimes do one thing, and sometimes another: e.g. in Year 8 Katy scores 1½ for her journey to school, because she sometimes goes by car and sometimes goes by bus.)

   b   Explain which period of time on the graph is the best example of continuity.

   c   Does the rate of change vary? Explain your answer.

   d   Is there a trend? If so, explain what it is.

   e   Is there a turning point for either of them? If so, explain what it is.

   f   Explain what factors you think affected the changes in their journeys to and from school.

4   Make a timeline or a graph to show change in your life over time. Show any trends or turning points, and places where the rate of change increases. Explain what factors have influenced these changes.

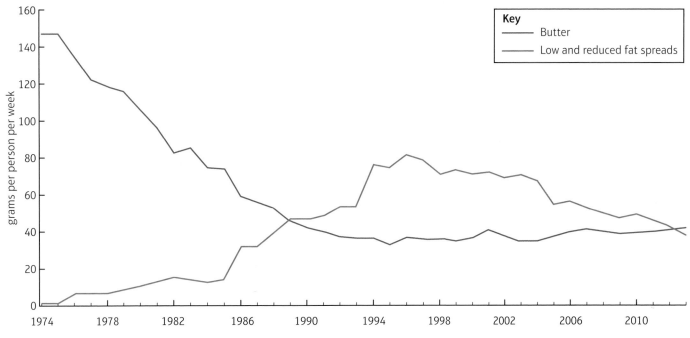

UK purchases of butter and spreads, 1974–2013

Journeys to and from school

School year	Katy	Mel
Years 1–6	Mel and Katy are twins; they went to a primary school that was about 10 minutes walk from home. Their Dad walked with them to school in the morning, and their Mum met them and walked home with them at the end of the day.	
Year 7	They now moved to a secondary school which was about three miles away. Their Mum took them to school in the car in the morning. They went to an after school club, and then their Dad picked them up in the car at about 5 o'clock.	
Year 8	Going to school, usually got a lift from her Mum in the car, but sometimes caught the bus with Mel and her friends. Stayed at the after school club until Dad picked them up in the car.	Caught the bus to school with her friends. Stayed at the after school club until Dad picked them up in the car.
Year 9	Cycled to school with her mates Aarav and Claire. Often stayed to do sport after school, and then cycled home.	Caught the bus to school with her friends. Usually stayed at the after school club until her Dad picked her up in the car. In the summer sometimes went home on the bus with her friends.
Year 10	Cycled to school with her mates. Often stayed to do sport after school, and then cycled home. In the summer developed a crush on one of Mel's friends, Callum, and started going in on the bus with Mel and her friends.	Caught the bus to school with her friends. Went home on the bus with her friends.
Year 11	Started going out with Callum. Usually met him on the bus in the mornings, and walked home with him after school.	Caught the bus to school with her friends. Went home on the bus with her friends.

Timeline: Medicine

Late Middle Ages	Tudor	Stuart

Ideas about causes and prevention

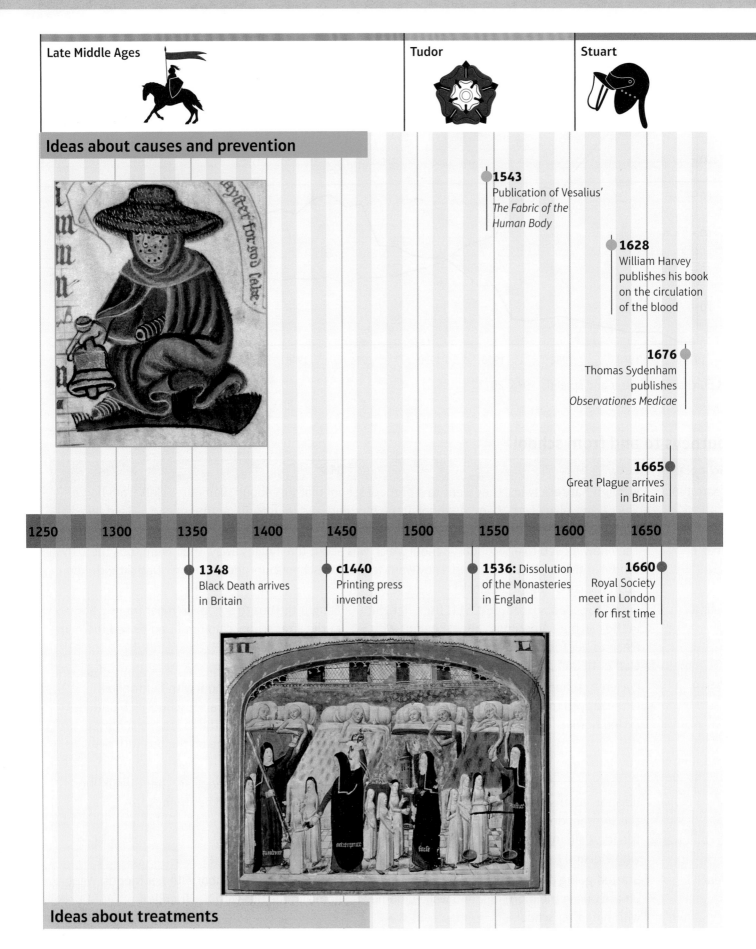

1543
Publication of Vesalius'
*The Fabric of the
Human Body*

1628
William Harvey
publishes his book
on the circulation
of the blood

1676
Thomas Sydenham
publishes
Observationes Medicae

1665
Great Plague arrives
in Britain

1250   1300   1350   1400   1450   1500   1550   1600   1650

1348
Black Death arrives
in Britain

c1440
Printing press
invented

1536: Dissolution
of the Monasteries
in England

1660
Royal Society
meet in London
for first time

Ideas about treatments

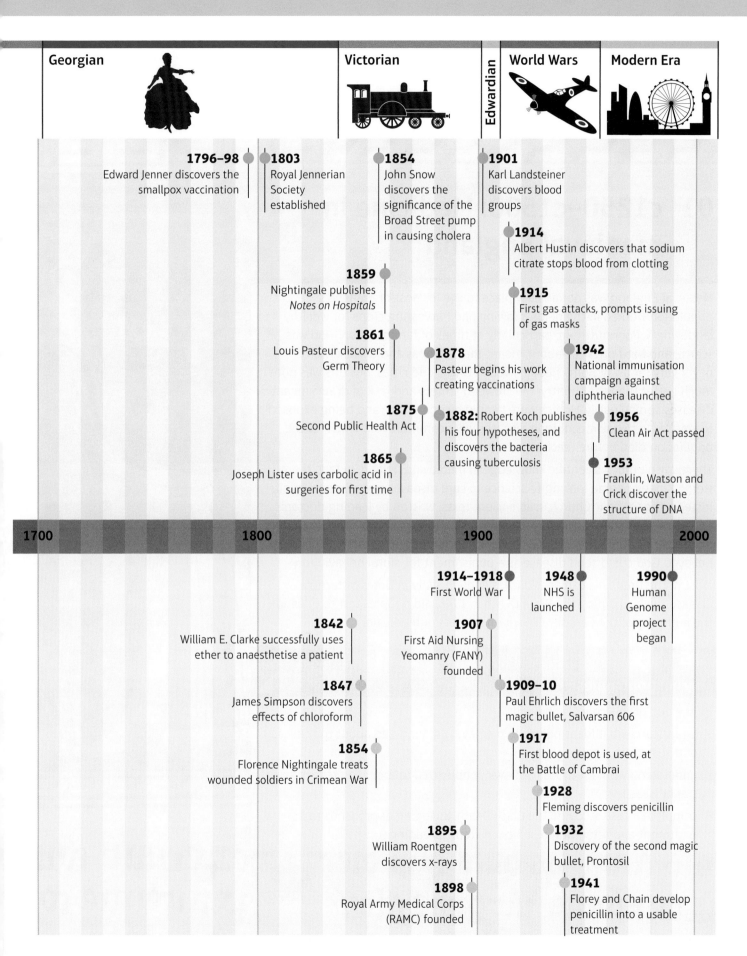

Georgian	Victorian	Edwardian	World Wars	Modern Era

1796–98
Edward Jenner discovers the smallpox vaccination

1803
Royal Jennerian Society established

1854
John Snow discovers the significance of the Broad Street pump in causing cholera

1901
Karl Landsteiner discovers blood groups

1914
Albert Hustin discovers that sodium citrate stops blood from clotting

1859
Nightingale publishes *Notes on Hospitals*

1915
First gas attacks, prompts issuing of gas masks

1861
Louis Pasteur discovers Germ Theory

1878
Pasteur begins his work creating vaccinations

1942
National immunisation campaign against diphtheria launched

1875
Second Public Health Act

1882: Robert Koch publishes his four hypotheses, and discovers the bacteria causing tuberculosis

1956
Clean Air Act passed

1865
Joseph Lister uses carbolic acid in surgeries for first time

1953
Franklin, Watson and Crick discover the structure of DNA

1700　　**1800**　　**1900**　　**2000**

1914–1918
First World War

1948
NHS is launched

1990
Human Genome project began

1842
William E. Clarke successfully uses ether to anaesthetise a patient

1907
First Aid Nursing Yeomanry (FANY) founded

1847
James Simpson discovers effects of chloroform

1909–10
Paul Ehrlich discovers the first magic bullet, Salvarsan 606

1917
First blood depot is used, at the Battle of Cambrai

1854
Florence Nightingale treats wounded soldiers in Crimean War

1928
Fleming discovers penicillin

1895
William Roentgen discovers x-rays

1932
Discovery of the second magic bullet, Prontosil

1898
Royal Army Medical Corps (RAMC) founded

1941
Florey and Chain develop penicillin into a usable treatment

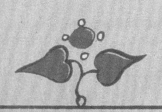

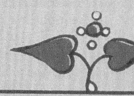
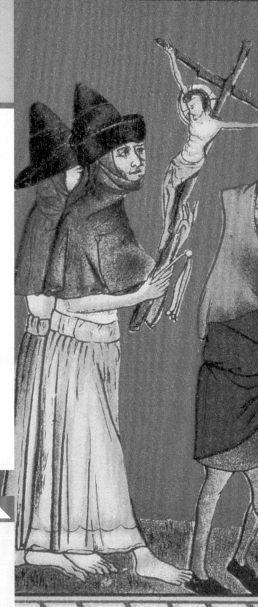

01 | c1250–c1500: Medicine in medieval England

Medieval England was not an easy place to live in. Most of England's population worked in the fields, growing and harvesting crops for wealthy landowners. Poor nutrition, particularly at times of famine when food was scarce, and hard physical labour, meant that sickness and disease were never very far away. Some people lived in towns and cities, but this was not much better than the country: the crowded streets and lack of drains meant diseases spread easily. Homes were heated by open fires, and being exposed to smoke every day meant lung diseases were common. Nearly half of the population died before reaching adulthood.

There wasn't much scientific knowledge in medieval England. In fact, there weren't many people looking to science to cure diseases and ailments at all. Instead, the Catholic Church used ancient texts, written by leading doctors and physicians such as Hippocrates and Galen, to explain why people caught diseases – or they said it was God's will when somebody became ill. People believed God could send disease as a punishment for sinful behaviour.

Most of the time, this explanation was enough. Only in times of terrible disease, such as during the Black Death in 1348, did people start to question the authority of the Catholic Church on matters of medicine.

Learning outcomes

By the end of this chapter, you will:

- understand what ideas people in medieval England had about the causes of disease and illness
- understand what methods medieval people tried in order to prevent and treat disease
- complete a case study on the Black Death, including approaches to its treatment and attempts to prevent it from spreading.

Learning outcomes

- Understand different ideas about the cause of disease before 1500, including the Theory of the Four Humours.
- Know the different influences on ideas about the cause of disease before 1500.

Supernatural and religious explanations of the causes of disease

Source A

The devil, or Satan, was often held responsible for sending diseases to people. This picture is taken from a 12th-century manuscript. In the image, Satan is infecting Job. According to the Bible, Job was very obedient and faithful to God. Satan argued that he was only faithful because his life was so good. Infecting him with a disease was used to test his faith.

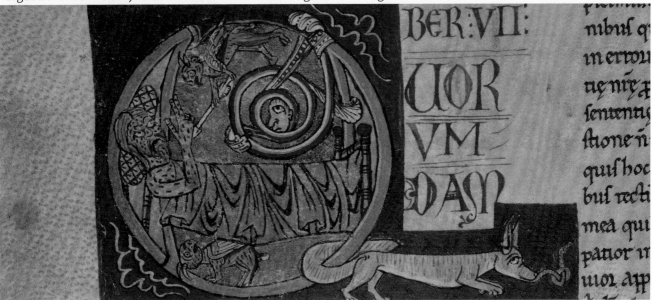

People in medieval England were very religious. The vast majority of people in England followed the teachings of the Catholic Church. They attended services regularly and were expected to give a sum of money to the Church each month. This was known as a **tithe**. The Church also owned large amounts of land in England, where it built churches, monasteries and convents. These became important centres of the community: as well as praying, monks and nuns of the Church provided basic medical care, looking after people who were not able to care for themselves. The Church used the tithes given by ordinary people to pay for the care of the community.

Illness was not uncommon. Malnutrition*, particularly in times of famine*, made people more likely to fall ill. A lack of scientific knowledge at this time meant that the causes of disease and illness were a mystery. The Church used religion to answer the questions people had about illness and disease.

Ordinary people received most of their teaching from the Church, as they didn't receive any formal education. The majority of people at this time could not read or write. Instead, they learned from the stories they heard, or the paintings they saw on the wall of their church. One thing they learned was that sin was very dangerous. The Church taught that those who committed a sin could be punished by God. They also taught that the devil could send disease to test someone's faith, as seen in Source A.

Key terms

Malnutrition*

An illness caused by lack of food.

Famine*

Food shortage, usually due to bad harvests.

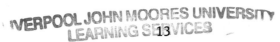

The Church often explained famine by saying that God had sent it as a punishment for sin. Therefore, it was logical also to blame people's sins for their illnesses. This meant that, when people recovered, the Church was able to declare that a miracle had happened, thanks to the patient's prayers. Therefore, blaming sickness on God acted as 'proof of the divine': it provided evidence of God's existence. This explains why the Church supported the idea that God sent disease as a punishment.

Although disease was mainly seen as a result of sin, the Church also taught that disease was sent by God to cleanse one's soul of sin. If you became ill, God could be sending the illness to purify your soul, or to test your faith. Since they had learned that God controlled every aspect of the world, this was very believable to people at this time.

Leprosy

The Bible tells many stories of how God sent disease as a punishment – leprosy in particular was included in the Bible as an illustration of a punishment for sin. Leprosy usually began as a painful skin disease, followed by paralysis* and eventually death. Fingers and toes would fall off, body hair would drop out and ulcers would develop both inside and outside the body.

Key term

Paralysis*

Being unable to move either all or part of your body as a result of illness, poison or injury.

There was no cure for leprosy, so lepers were banished from their communities. They usually had to move to leper houses or to isolated island communities. If they were allowed to stay in their home towns, they had to wear a cloak and ring a bell to announce their presence, and they were banned from going down narrow alleys, where it was impossible to avoid them.

Source B

A painting of a leper from around 1400. Lepers were made to wear a cloak to cover their diseased bodies and ring a bell to warn people when they were nearby. The bell would also have acted as a way to ask for alms, or charitable donations. The words say, 'Some good, my gentle master, for God's sake'.

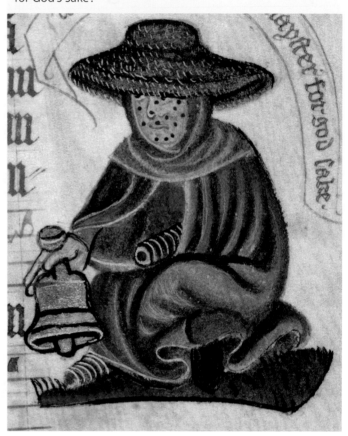

This was because it was believed their breath was contagious. Although this was not true (leprosy was spread only by very close contact with the infected), it does show that medieval people had some correct ideas about how some diseases were transmitted.

Although there was no formal care for lepers, a few **lazar** houses did help people suffering from leprosy. Lazar houses were more commonly known as leper colonies.

Astrology

Along with the role of God, the alignment of the planets and stars was also considered very important when diagnosing* illness. A physician* would consult star charts, looking at when the patient was born and when they fell ill, to help identify what was wrong.

Traditionally, the Church frowned upon the idea of using astrology in diagnosing illness, as it seemed only one step away from predicting the future, or fortune telling. However, after the Black Death arrived, astrology became more popular and the Church became more acceptant of it. Many people believed the Black Death was caused by a bad alignment of the planets.

Astrology was a **supernatural** explanation for disease. During the period c1250–c1500, the impact of the stars and planets on health was considered important because of the influence of Hippocrates (see page 17), who had been a leading physician from Ancient Greece.

The Theory of the Four Humours

Not all explanations for disease were supernatural or religious. A very popular idea, first put forwards by the Ancient Greeks, was the **Theory of the Four Humours**.

The theory stated that, as the universe was made up of the four basic elements – fire, water, earth and air – the body must also be made up of four humours, which were all created by digesting different foods. The four humours were:

- **blood**
- **phlegm** – the watery substance coughed up or sneezed out of the nose, or expelled in tears
- **black bile** – not one particular substance in the body, but probably referred to clotted blood, visible in excrement or vomit
- **choler**, or yellow bile – this appeared in pus or vomit.

There was a belief that all the humours must be balanced and equal. If the mix became unbalanced, you became ill. Being careful to maintain a good balance of the humours was really important to preserving good health. However, people believed a combination of age, family traits and circumstances, such as the season in which someone was born, usually combined to make one or two of the humours stronger than the others.

Key terms

Diagnosing*

Deciding what is wrong with a patient by considering different symptoms. In medieval England, physicians could also consider star charts to diagnose an illness.

Physician*

Someone who practices medicine. A medieval physician did not have to have the same level of training as a modern physician.

Activities

1 Draw a rough outline of a church building. Inside it, list at least three reasons why many people in the Middle Ages believed that the main cause of illness and disease was punishment from God.

2 Write a leaflet in the style of a medieval manuscript, offering advice on how to avoid disease and illness.

3 If people believed that God sent disease, what sort of treatments do you think they tried? Make a list – you can see how many you correctly predicted in the next section.

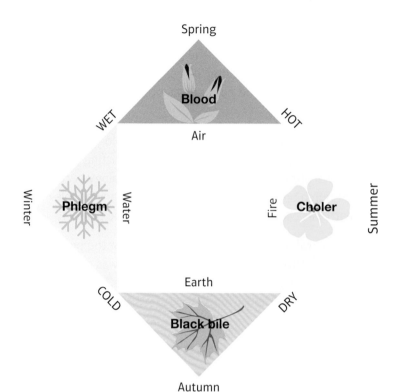

Figure 1.1 The Four Humours.

Humour	Season	Element	Qualities	Ancient name
Blood	Spring	Air	Hot and wet	Sanguine
Choler	Summer	Fire	Hot and dry	Choleric
Black bile	Autumn	Earth	Cold and dry	Melancholic
Phlegm	Winter	Water	Cold and wet	Phlegmatic

Activity ?

Create a paper fortune teller to help you remember the different parts of the Theory of the Four Humours.

a   On the outside, write the names of the four humours.

b   On the first layer inside, write the characteristics of each humour – hot, cold, wet, dry.

c   On the next layer, write anything else that is related to the humour – characteristics, seasons and star signs.

According to the theory, each humour was linked to certain characteristics that physicians would look for when carrying out their diagnosis. For example, a person suffering from a fever had a temperature, causing the skin to go hot and red because, physicians believed, they had too much blood. This was a hot and wet element. Meanwhile, a person suffering from a cold had too much phlegm, which was cold and wet. They would shiver and the excess phlegm would run out of their nose.

The humours were linked with the seasons. For example, in winter, which is cold and wet, it was thought that the body produces too much phlegm, causing coughs and colds as the patient tries to get rid of it. The star signs for each season were associated with its humour, too: Capricorn, Aquarius and Pisces were linked with phlegm. Astrology was considered an important part of the Theory of the Four Humours, as the humours were connected with star signs and seasons, and each one had its own ruling planet.

The humours were also linked with certain personality traits. For example, a quick tempered, argumentative person was said to have choleric characteristics, while an optimistic, calm person had cheerful tendencies (sanguine). What we would today recognise as depression was blamed on an excess of black bile (melancholic) in medieval times.

The origins of the theory

The Theory of the Four Humours was created by an Ancient Greek physician named Hippocrates in the 5th century BCE. The word 'humour' comes from the Greek word for fluid – humon. Hippocrates was very careful to observe all the **symptoms** of his patients and record them. The Theory of the Four Humours fitted with what he saw.

Galen, a physician in Ancient Rome during the 2nd century CE, liked the ideas of Hippocrates and developed them further. He had been a physician in a gladiator school and later became the personal physician of the Roman Emperor. This meant that he had lots of time to experiment, ponder philosophy and write. By the time he died, he left behind a very large body of work – more than 350 books.

If you are suffering from too much…

phlegm   blood

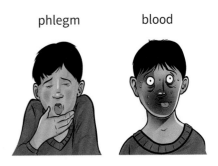

…then treatment is something…

hot and dry   cold and wet

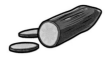

Figure 1.2 Examples of the Theory of Opposites.

Extend your knowledge

Galen's character
Galen had a reputation for being quite arrogant and a 'know-it-all'. He wrote about this in his works, using himself as an example of how one humour could be more dominant than another. He claimed that he had a naturally choleric temperament, which made him short-tempered. He thought he had inherited this from his mother, who was so bad tempered that she used to bite her servants!

Galen developed the Theory of the Four Humours to include the idea of balancing the humours by using the **Theory of Opposites**. For example, he suggested that too much phlegm, which was linked to water and the cold, could be cured by eating hot peppers; a fever, or an excess of blood, could be treated with cucumber, which would cool the patient down when eaten. Galen also theorised that the circulatory system circulated blood generated in the liver, and the blood was then distributed around the body.

Why was the theory so popular?

The Theory of the Four Humours was very detailed and could be used to explain away almost any kind of illness – physical or mental. It was important that the theory covered almost every type of illness that occurred, because there was no other scientific explanation for the cause of disease. Often, physicians twisted what they saw to fit with the logic of the theory.

Activities ?

1 Create an advice poster to explain how the Four Humours led to illness. Make sure you give examples of different illnesses caused by different imbalances.
2 Hippocrates and Galen were both physicians who had a huge impact on medieval medicine. Write a short paragraph to summarise their ideas and explain how Galen built on the work of Hippocrates.

Classical thinking in the Middle Ages

Hippocrates and Galen were both very popular figures in medieval medicine. Although written in the time of Ancient Greece and Rome, Latin translations of their texts only started to appear in Europe from the 11th century – almost 800 years after they were written. These translations were copied and recopied by monks, who passed them on to new medical universities. The first European medical school had been established in Salerno in the 9th century, and taught students based on these texts, rather than practical experience.

Extend your knowledge

The *Articella*

By the mid 13th century, medical students in European universities relied on the *Articella* to tell them everything they needed to know about medicine. This medical textbook included some directly translated works from Hippocrates and Galen. It also included the work of a 9th-century Persian doctor, Hunayn ibn-Is'haq, who had studied the work of both Hippocrates and Galen.

Other classical works were also popular among physicians and medical students, including those of the Greek thinker, Aristotle, and the Persian philosopher and physician, Avicenna. Physicians were expected to have a good background in the liberal arts, such as philosophy, before studying medicine.

Galen's influence

However, classical texts like those of Galen continued to be very influential in the Middle Ages for three reasons: the influence of the Church, the importance of book learning and the lack of alternative theories.

The influence of the Church

Galen wrote that the body was clearly designed for a purpose and that the different parts of the body were meant to work together in balance, as first proposed by Hippocrates. Galen also believed in the idea of the soul. This theory fitted in very well with the ideas of the Church, who believed that God created man in his image, and so they promoted Galen's teachings and, by extension, those of Hippocrates. Since books were produced in monasteries, and libraries were maintained by the Church, their choice of texts were the ones that were widely read, preached and believed. In the early Middle Ages, the Church controlled medical learning in universities, too.

The importance of book learning

Many people could not read in the Middle Ages. This meant that being widely read was a sign of intelligence. A good physician was considered to be one who had read many books, rather than one who had treated a lot of patients. Having read the works of Hippocrates and Galen was proof that a physician was worth the money he was being paid. The authority of these classical texts was so strong that people believed them even when there was actual, physical evidence that suggested they were wrong.

The lack of alternatives

There was a lack of scientific evidence to support any other kind of theories of the causes of disease. Dissections were mostly illegal, because the Church taught that the body needed to be buried whole in order for the soul to go to heaven. Very occasionally, physicians were able to dissect executed criminals, or criminals who had been sentenced to death by vivisection*. When this happened, the physician would sit far away from the body, reading from the works of Galen, while the actual cutting and examining was done by a barber surgeon*. This meant that Galen's ideas were preserved: anything in the body that didn't agree with Galen's writings could be explained away, since the body was that of a criminal and therefore imperfect, and the physician himself never did any of the examinations.

Key terms

Vivisection*

Criminals sentenced to death by vivisection had their bodies cut open (dissected) and examined by physicians and medical students.

Barber surgeon*

Barbers worked with sharp knives, so as well as giving people haircuts, they also carried out medical procedures such as blood-letting (see page 23). Over time, they took on smaller surgeries.

Exam-style question, Section B

Explain why there was continuity in ideas about the cause of disease during the period c1250–c1500.

You may use the following information in your answer:

* the Church
* Galen.

You **must** also use information of your own.   **12 marks**

Exam tip

There are **six marks** available here for your knowledge and **six marks** available for how well you explain your answer.

* Make sure you use your **own knowledge** as well as what is suggested by the bullet points. If you don't, you are limiting yourself to a maximum of eight marks.
* Think about **structure** and **coherence**. Before you start writing, think carefully about the order of your points and make links between them.

Source C

A picture of a medieval dissection. The physician is sitting high up, away from the body. He is reading aloud from the works of Galen. The body is being dissected by somebody else. This painting appeared in the first illustrated anatomy book to be printed – the *Fasciculus Medicinae*, written by Joannes de Ketham, an Austrian professor of medicine, in 1491.

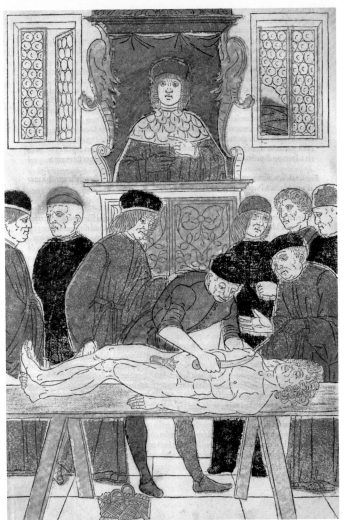

Other ideas about the cause of disease

Miasma

A **miasma** was bad air that was believed to be filled with harmful fumes. Hippocrates and Galen both wrote about miasmata (which is the plural of miasma) and suggested that swamps, corpses and other rotting matter could transmit disease.

Extend your knowledge

The Romans

Over a thousand years before the 13th century, the Romans had built their settlements away from swamps and smelly places in an effort to avoid miasmic diseases, such as malaria. Indeed, the word malaria comes from the Italian words 'mala' – which means bad, and 'aria' – which means air.

Smells and vapours like miasmata were also, unsurprisingly, associated with God. A clean and sweet-smelling home was a sign of spiritual cleanliness, and incense was burned in churches to purify the air. Homes that smelled badly suggested sinfulness and corruption and, if a person was unwashed, other people would avoid them, in case they breathed in the bad miasma and contracted a disease. This was also why people avoided lepers. Although many believed leprosy was a punishment from God, they also believed the disease was contagious.

Extend your knowledge

More on miasma
It is worth noting that medieval physicians didn't use the word 'miasma' to describe disease-spreading air, as far as we can tell from the evidence we have. Instead, they referred to it as 'corruption of the air', 'pestilential air' or 'putrefaction of the air'. 'Miasma' was not used regularly until later.

Urine charts

Although medieval physicians didn't blame people's urine for making them ill, they did carefully examine the urine in order to make their diagnosis. It was thought to be one of the best ways to check on the balance of the humours inside the body. Samples of a patient's urine could be sent to a physician, where it would be examined and compared with a urine chart.

The physician would carefully check the colour, thickness, smell and even taste of the urine before making his diagnosis. This was seen as a very important part of medieval medicine: Norwich Cathedral Priory, for example, employed a full-time physician to examine urine.

Influences on ideas about the cause of disease

The Middle Ages was a time when there was **continuity** in ideas about the cause of disease. There were only a few small changes. For example, the use of astrology became more widespread, which meant it was adopted by many people, but did not expand upon Galen's original theories. On the whole, ideas remained the same.

Individuals and the Church

The Church was very important in maintaining the status quo at this time. This means that they did not like change, and wanted to keep things the way they were. The Church controlled medical learning. It chose which books were copied and distributed. The Church liked the Theory of the Four Humours because it fitted with their teachings, so it promoted this theory. The Church strongly discouraged anybody from criticising the theory.

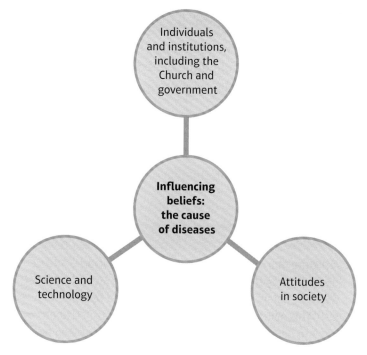

Figure 1.3 Three main factors to understanding change and continuity in early diagnosis of disease.

Hippocrates and Galen were important individuals in the Middle Ages, even though they lived many years before this time. Their books had been preserved by Arabic scholars and Latin translations were available in Europe by the Middle Ages. Galen in particular was popular with the Church, which meant that his work was widely promoted.

Science and technology

During the Middle Ages, a lack of scientific understanding meant that new knowledge was limited. Physicians and medical students tried to make new discoveries fit into the old theories, rather than experimenting to explain the discoveries.

One important piece of technology invented near the end of the Middle Ages was the **printing press**. It was invented in around 1440 by Johannes Gutenberg in what is now Germany. Although this was not directly related to advancing medieval medicine, it eventually led to much faster and easier sharing of medical texts. However, it did not have a huge impact during the medieval period.

Attitudes in society

Medieval people had a strong belief in God and did not want to risk going to hell by being critical of the Church. Physicians who did not follow the old ideas found it hard to get work, because everybody knew a 'good' physician would follow the Theory of the Four Humours. A famous 13th-century military surgeon, Henri de Mondeville, was among those who questioned the old ways of practising medicine. Mondeville is even quoted as stating that classical figures like Hippocrates and Galen were like an old dog that needed to be put down, but whose owner could not face replacing it with a younger, healthier dog. However, even he continued to practise medicine in the same way as everybody else – he probably wouldn't have found employment otherwise.

Many people believed that, since medicine had always been done this way, there was no need to change it.

Activity ?

This activity will help you to decide the importance of each key idea about the cause of illness in the years c1250–c1500.

a On slips of paper, write down the key ideas about the causes of illness at this time: God; imbalanced humours; miasma; alignment of the planets/stars.

b Now put these into a hierarchy. Which do you think was the most important? Which was the least important? Do we still believe any of them today? Were some of these ideas more important to particular groups of people, or at different times?

c Look back over the information in this section if you need to jog your memory. Discuss your ideas with another person or in a small group.

Summary

- Many people believed that disease was a punishment or test from God because of sin.
- The Theory of the Four Humours was very popular. It stated that an imbalance in the humours could cause illness.
- Other ideas about the causes of disease and illness included miasma (bad air) and a misalignment in the planets or stars.

Checkpoint

Strengthen

S1 Create a spider diagram or a bullet point list to show the different ideas people had between 1250 and 1500 about what caused illness and disease.

S2 List the four humours and their properties.

S3 Describe, in detail, the role of Hippocrates and Galen in medieval medicine.

Challenge

C1 Explain both **why** and **how** the Church had an impact on medieval medicine.

If you are not confident about this question, form a group with other students, discuss the answer and then record your conclusion. Your teacher can give you some hints.

1.2 Approaches to treatment and prevention

Religious and supernatural treatments

As the Church taught that disease was sent by God as a punishment for sin, it followed that the cure should also involve the supernatural. As well as looking for medical treatment for disease, it was important to undergo a course of spiritual healing. Religious treatments included:

• healing prayers and incantations (spells)
• paying for a special mass* to be said
• fasting (going without food).

Pilgrimages* to the tombs of people noted for their healing powers also became extremely popular. Once the pilgrimage was complete, there were a few suggested actions those with diseases could take (see Figure 1.4).

Key terms

Mass*

Roman Catholic service where bread and wine is given. Catholics believe that this involves a miracle: the bread and wine is turned into the body and blood of Christ.

Pilgrimage*

A journey to an important religious monument, shrine or place.

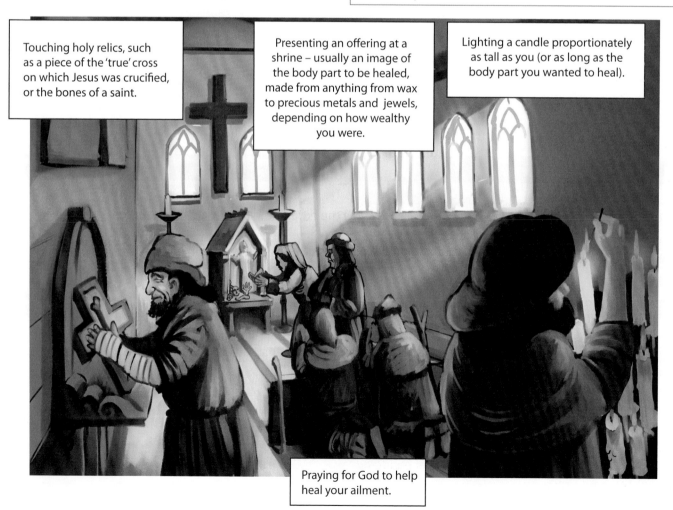

Touching holy relics, such as a piece of the 'true' cross on which Jesus was crucified, or the bones of a saint.

Presenting an offering at a shrine – usually an image of the body part to be healed, made from anything from wax to precious metals and jewels, depending on how wealthy you were.

Lighting a candle proportionately as tall as you (or as long as the body part you wanted to heal).

Praying for God to help heal your ailment.

Figure 1.4 Pilgrims suffering from disease visit a holy site.

As well as making the locals a lot of money, as the pilgrims brought with them money to spend in the towns of holy sites, the ability to heal the sick was also important to the local churchmen. In order to be declared a saint, the dead person had to be associated with a certain number of miracles; so, the more people who were 'healed' after touching the relics, the better.

Extend your knowledge

The king's healing power

It was widely believed that the king had the power to heal certain illnesses. During the coronation of a monarch, his hands would be rubbed with special holy oil and this, it was said, gave him supernatural healing powers. The king's touch was considered particularly effective for scrofula, a form of tuberculosis. Kings took this very seriously, as it was a good way to demonstrate their divine right (the idea that God had chosen them to be king). Edward I, for example, aimed to touch up to 2,000 people a year during his reign (1272–1307).

If prayers and offerings did not work, there were other supernatural remedies available, although the Church did not approve of them. Chanting incantations and using charms or amulets to heal symptoms and ward off diseases were fairly common throughout this period.

Sometimes the sick were discouraged from seeking cures. After all, if God had sent the disease to purge the soul, it was important for the disease to run its course. Taking medicine to cure the disease might keep you alive, but it would mean that your soul would still be stained with sin. That meant risking not being admitted into heaven when you died.

Astrology

Physicians consulted star charts when diagnosing illness. These were also important when prescribing treatment. Treatments varied according to the horoscope of the patient. The alignment of the planets was then checked at every stage of the treatment prescribed: herb gathering, bleeding, purging, operations and even cutting hair and nails all had to be done at the right time.

Humoural treatments

Today, when we fall ill, doctors assess the symptoms, make a diagnosis and treat the infection. For example, if a patient catches a chest infection, the treatment prescribed will be to attack the germ, rather than to stop the patient from coughing. This is because modern medicine recognises that treating the cause of the illness will eventually treat the symptom.

Medieval physicians did not work in the same way. Each symptom was broken down and treated separately, as they believed each symptom represented an imbalance in the humours. Therefore, conflicting remedies might be provided.

Source A

Advice from John of Gaddesden's medical book, the *Rosa Anglica*. John, a very well-respected English physician, wrote this very popular medical text in the 14th century. Here, he explains how to cure lethargy [extreme tiredness].

It is necessary for lethargics that people talk loudly in their presence. Tie their extremities lightly and rub their palms and soles hard; and let their feet be put in salt water up to the middle of their shins, and pull their hair and nose, and squeeze the toes and fingers tightly, and cause pigs to squeal in their ears; give them a sharp clyster [an enema] at the beginning… and open the vein of the head, or nose, or forehead, and draw blood from the nose with the bristles of a boar. Put a feather, or a straw, in his nose to compel him to sneeze, and do not ever desist from hindering him from sleeping; and let human hair or other evil-smelling thing be burnt under his nose…

Blood-letting

Phlebotomy, or blood-letting/bleeding, was the most common treatment for an imbalance in the humours. The idea behind it was that bad humours could be removed from the body by removing some of the blood.

Phlebotomy was so common that most physicians didn't even bother to carry out the procedure themselves – and monks were forbidden from bleeding their patients.

Instead, it was usually done by barber surgeons and wise women. Demand was so high that even some people with no medical background offered the service.

Bleeding was carried out in several different ways.

Type	Method	Uses
Cutting a vein	This involved cutting open a vein with a lancet or other sharp instrument. Blood was usually let from a vein near the elbow, because it was easy to access.	The most straightforward method of bleeding. Phlebotomy charts like the vein man (see Source B) were used to show points in the body where bleeding was recommended for specific illnesses.
Leeches	Freshwater leeches were collected, washed and kept hungry for a day before being placed on the skin. Bleeding might continue for up to 10 hours after the leech was full.	Used for people whose age or condition made traditional bleeding too dangerous.
Cupping	The skin was pierced with a knife or a pin, or even scratched with fingernails, until it was bleeding. A heated cup was placed over the cuts to create a vacuum. This drew blood out of the skin.	Used for women, children and the very old. People believed different areas treated different illnesses. For example, people believed that cupping on the back of the neck was good for eye trouble, bad breath and facial acne.

Sometimes patients were bled for too long and died as a result. Evidence suggests that this was quite common and it was probably seen as a necessary hazard. In 1278, court records from an inquest in London show that William le Paumer had collapsed and died due to a blood-letting procedure that had taken place the previous day. The court did not hold anybody responsible for the death, and didn't even name the person who had carried out the bleeding.

Source B

A vein man, or phlebotomy chart. This picture was printed in a manual belonging to the York Barbers in the late 15th century. It shows points on the body where blood-letting should happen, matching different ailments with different places on the body. For example, if a patient was suffering from depression, the recommendation was to bleed them from a vein in the back.

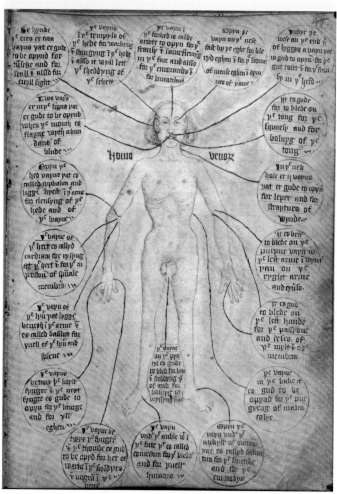

Purging

Because it was believed that the humours were created from the foods eaten, a common treatment was purging the digestive system to remove any leftover food. This was done by giving the patient either something to make them vomit (an emetic), or a laxative or enema to clear out anything left over in the body.

Emetics usually consisted of strong and bitter herbs like scammony, aniseed and parsley. Sometimes they contained poisons like black hellebore, so it was best to vomit them up quickly.

Laxatives were very common. Some well-known examples included mallow leaves stewed in ale, and linseeds fried in hot fat. Linseeds are still used today as a digestive aid.

Sometimes people needed a bit more help to purge, and the physician would administer a **clyster** or enema. For example, John of Arderne, a famous English surgeon, mixed water with honey, oil, wheat bran, soap and herbs such as mallow and camomile. He would squirt it into the patient's anus using a greased pipe fixed to a pig's bladder, while the patient rubbed his stomach. This would clear out any stubborn blockages.

Remedies

Sick people in the period c1250–c1500 were also treated with remedies – usually herbal infusions to drink, sniff or bathe in.

Some of these are still in use today. For example, aloe vera was prescribed to improve digestion. Other ingredients featured regularly included mint, camomile and rose oils, tamarind, almonds, saffron, butter, absinth, turpentine and corals. Sometimes the ingredients were expensive and difficult to find.

A common remedy mixed and sold at this time was **theriaca**. This was a spice-based mixture that could contain up to 70 ingredients, including quite common things like ginger, cardamom, pepper and saffron, but also some unusual ingredients like viper flesh and opium. Galen had written a book on theriacas, looking particularly at their use in treating snake bites and poisons. Over time, they became widely popular and were used for many different illnesses.

Different foods were prescribed to encourage the balance of the humours – remember that the humours were thought to be created from the digestion of food. A dish called **blanc mangier**, made from chicken and almonds, was regularly recommended for medieval invalids because the ingredients were warm and moist.

Bathing

Warm baths were regularly prescribed to help the body draw in heat to help dissolve blockages in the humours. This gave the body the opportunity to steam out impurities and ease aching joints. Herbal remedies could also be given this way.

Various plants and herbs were added to the bath water to help. For example, people suffering from bladder stones were advised to stir in mallow and violets.

Some of the remedies were less pleasant and were based purely on superstition: those suffering from paralysis were advised to boil a fox in water and then bathe in it! This was because it was thought that the quick and nimble properties of the fox would be transferred to the patient through the bath water.

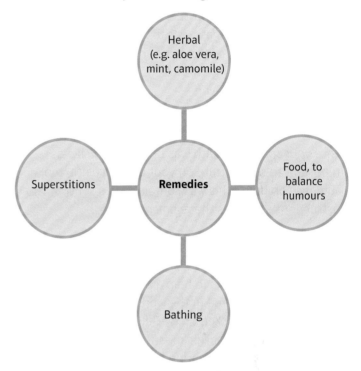

Figure 1.5 Common remedies, c1250–c1500.

Preventing disease

Although a physician could expect to be paid a lot more money for providing treatments for disease, there was a strong focus on following various regimes to prevent getting sick in the first place. This was seen as a far safer plan of action, since cures and treatments were hit-and-miss in their effectiveness.

The Church

Most people believed that the best, and most important, way of preventing disease was to lead a life free from sin. Regular prayers, confessions and offering tithes to the Church worked together to ensure that any minor sins were quickly forgiven.

Hygiene

Once your spiritual health was taken care of, it was important to concentrate on your bodily health, too. Guidance on doing this was contained in a set of instructions known as the *regimen sanitatis*.

Regimen Sanitatis

The *regimen sanitatis* was a loose set of instructions provided by physicians to help a patient maintain good health. It first appeared in the work of Hippocrates, where it was later picked up by Galen and Arabic scholars like Avicenna. This meant that the advice was widespread and very common by 1250. A lot of the advice is familiar to us today.

Ideally, a physician would provide a regimen sanitatis written especially for their patient, taking into account their predominant humours and lifestyle. However, in practice, this service was only used by the very rich, because it took a long time to write such a detailed set of instructions for every patient.

Bathing was an important treatment for disease. It was also used as a preventative measure: bad smells indicated a miasma. However, only the wealthy could afford a private bath of hot water. Public baths, or **stewes**, were available for a fee. Poorer people swam in rivers, where possible, to keep themselves fresh. Although only the wealthy bathed their whole bodies regularly, everybody – no matter how poor – washed their hands before and usually after every meal. They believed that cleanliness was next to godliness, so it was important to stay clean.

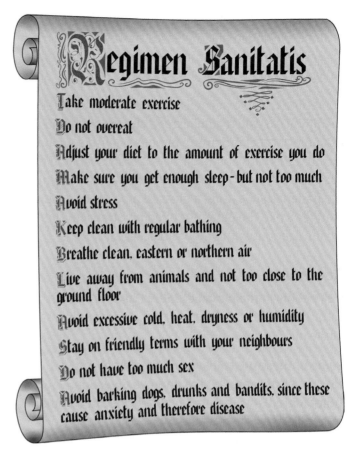

Regimen Sanitatis

Take moderate exercise

Do not overeat

Adjust your diet to the amount of exercise you do

Make sure you get enough sleep – but not too much

Avoid stress

Keep clean with regular bathing

Breathe clean, eastern or northern air

Live away from animals and not too close to the ground floor

Avoid excessive cold, heat, dryness or humidity

Stay on friendly terms with your neighbours

Do not have too much sex

Avoid barking dogs, drunks and bandits, since these cause anxiety and therefore disease

Figure 1.6 Advice given in the *regimen sanitatis*.

As well as keeping themselves clean, people also tried to make sure their homes smelled sweet and fresh, too. Floors were swept regularly and rushes were laid down to soak up any mess. Sometimes sweet smelling herbs, like lavender, were spread with the rushes to keep the air free of miasmata.

Diet

Since the humours were thought to be produced by digestion, what and when you ate were both considered very important in preventing an imbalance. Eating too much was strongly discouraged.

According to the chroniclers of the time, several medieval kings died as a result of eating too much, or having too rich a diet. Edward I died of dysentery*, for example.

Key term
Dysentery*
Very severe diarrhoea.

Fear of digestive problems leading to death was so great that many people purged themselves, either by vomiting or using laxatives, as a way of preventing disease as well as treating it. Hippocrates recommended using an emetic once a fortnight in the winter, and to use enemas in the summer.

Purifying the air

Medieval people attempted to keep the air free from miasmata by purifying it. They did this by spreading sweet herbs, such as lavender. Sometimes this might be carried as a bunch of flowers (posy), or placed inside a decorative piece of jewellery called a pomander (a large locket, which would be worn around the waist).

Local authorities, usually under the direction of magistrates or noblemen, also tried to tackle miasmata outside of the home, putting into place measures to keep towns clean. For example, they tried to make sure there were no rotting animals left lying around and pulled down or cleaned particularly smelly public toilets.

Medieval 'medics'

Most people in the Middle Ages would have been treated at home by a female family member. Women did most of the treatment at home, caring for the sick and mixing remedies themselves. Women also acted as midwives: evidence from medieval sources suggests that only women attended births.

Asking for medical advice cost a lot of money. Since the treatments weren't guaranteed, most people were not willing to spend this money even if they had it. However, there were other treatment options for people willing to pay.

Physicians

During the Middle Ages, new universities were set up across Europe, including Oxford, Cambridge, Paris, Bologna, Montpellier and Padua. Medicine became more professional. A medical degree took between seven and ten years to complete, depending on the level and university.

Medieval doctors were known as physicians – the word 'doctor' did not become common until the 17th century.

The main role of a physician was to diagnose illness and recommend a course of treatment. They rarely got involved in treating the patients themselves – this was left up to less educated midwives, apothecaries or barber surgeons.

If you were lucky enough to be able to afford a physician, he might attend in person to examine you, but this wasn't really considered necessary. The consultation would follow three stages.

1 The physician would look at a sample of the patient's urine, faeces and blood, all of which would be collected and sent to him.

2 He would also consult the astrological charts under which the patient was born and at the time they fell sick.

3 Based on this, and the humoural tendencies of the patient (whether they were naturally sanguine, choleric, phlegmatic or melancholic), the physician would create a course of treatment.

It was then up to less trained and lower paid professionals to carry out the treatment. For most of this period, this was due to the fact that many physicians were clergymen, who were forbidden from carrying out procedures such as bleeding. From 1215 onwards, any operations likely to involve cutting the patient were also forbidden for clergymen.

During this time, new universities and centres for medical learning were set up in Europe without religious sponsorship. Foreign physicians who had no connection to the Church were able to both diagnose and treat their patients.

Physicians were very expensive, because there weren't many of them. This was mainly due to the training taking a long time. Royalty and the very wealthy often employed a physician full time. Others paid for them when they needed them.

Apothecaries

Apothecaries mainly mixed herbal remedies. They had a good knowledge of the healing power of herbs and plants thanks to studying herbal manuals such as *Materia Medica*. They usually had a good amount of knowledge from their own experience, or passed down from family members.

Apothecaries were not considered as skilled or knowledgeable as physicians. Physicians prescribed the medication and apothecaries were just there to mix the remedy. However, since doctors were expensive and apothecaries were comparatively cheap, lots of people would see an apothecary as an alternative to a doctor. This meant that doctors saw them as a threat to their livelihood.

Source C

A picture of an apothecary's shop taken from an Italian medical text published in the 14th century. The shelves are filled with large, ornate jars, which held theriac.

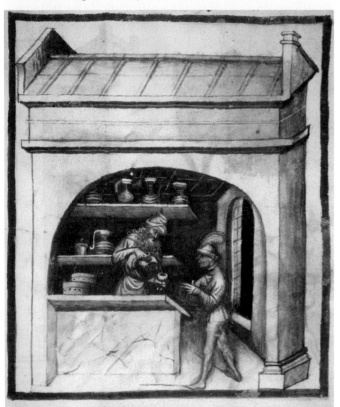

Apothecaries did not just create remedies, they also prescribed poison. This went against an idea fundamental to physicians – that they should do no harm. This rule went all the way back to Hippocrates and still exists today: all doctors must swear a Hippocratic Oath before practising medicine. Apothecaries were not bound by this rule, so they could not be trusted to do the best for their patient. Nor did they need to attend university to set up their business.

Finally, many apothecaries also dabbled in alchemy and the supernatural, providing amulets and charms for patients who wanted something extra to cure a disease. This was frowned upon by the Church and, since many physicians were also priests, this meant that the gap between physicians and apothecaries became even wider.

Surgeons

Barber surgeons were probably the least qualified medical professionals in England. Since good barbers had sharp knives and a steady hand, they regularly performed small surgeries as well, such as pulling teeth and bleeding patients.

Extend your knowledge

Barber surgeons

Until 1307, barber surgeons advertised their services by putting a bowl of blood in their shop windows; after that, they displayed the sign of a bandaged, bloodied arm, which later became the red and white striped barber pole still used today.

Some surgeons were highly trained: in Europe, some physicians were encouraged to study surgery alongside medicine, so many learned their skills at university. In fact, the quality of surgery was arguably higher than the quality of medical advice, because it was usually based on experience rather than knowledge learned from books. In medieval England, a skilled surgeon could set a broken limb, remove an arrow or even successfully remove cataracts from the eyes.

Activities ?

1 Draw a cartoon stick figure to represent each different medical professional. Add labels to explain what sort of treatments each person carried out.

2 Explain how each of the different professionals was trained to do their job.

3 Why do you think there was so much friction between the different types of medics in medieval England?

Caring for the sick: hospitals and the home

Hospitals

The number of hospitals in England was on the rise during the Middle Ages. By 1500, there were an estimated 1,100 hospitals, ranging in size from just a few beds to hundreds. Bury St Edmund's, for example, had at least six hospitals to cater for lepers, the infirm and the old. The city had a shrine famous for its healing powers and therefore attracted a lot of sick people. However, many hospitals did not actually treat the sick. Instead, they offered **hospitality** to travellers and pilgrims, which is how hospitals got their name.

About 30% of the hospitals in England were owned and run by the Church in the Middle Ages. These were run by the monks and nuns who lived in nearby monasteries.

The rest were funded by an **endowment**, where a wealthy person had left money in their will for the setting up of a hospital. Since charity was a foundation of religion and the Church taught that charitable donations could help to heal disease, it is not surprising that there were so many. The Church was in charge of running many of these hospitals, too.

Medieval hospitals that did treat the sick were not the same as the hospitals we have today.

Medieval hospitals were good places to rest and recover. The space would have been kept very clean and the bed linens and clothing of the patients changed regularly. It was a large part of the nuns' duties to do the washing and make sure everywhere was kept clean. This meant that, for people not suffering from terminal disease, hospitals were probably quite successful.

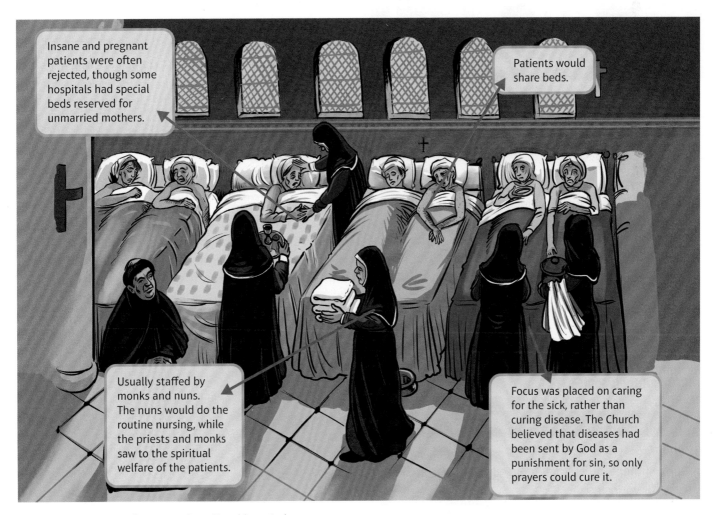

Figure 1.7 Common features of medieval hospitals.

Source D

A picture of a medieval hospital, from 1482. Some of the patients are sharing beds, which was normal at this time. The only patient allowed their own bed was a dying woman. Henry VII's famous hospital, the Savoy, opened in 1512. It was unique in offering all patients their own beds.

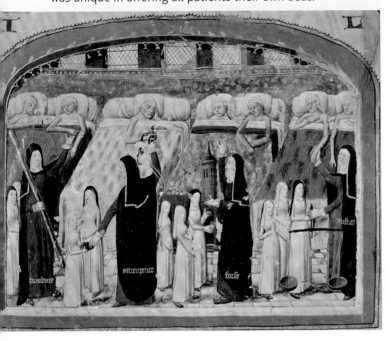

Naturally, this is what the Church wanted: a recovery was further proof of the existence of God and the importance of prayer.

Many European hospitals employed physicians and surgeons, but there is no evidence to suggest that English hospitals did the same. Since religious men were forbidden from cutting into the body, treatment was very limited.

Infectious or terminal patients were often rejected from hospitals, as prayer and penance* could do nothing for these people. However, patients who had a chance of recovery were able to see the altar and even participate in Church services from their beds, to help with the healing of their souls.

Key term

Penance*

A punishment inflicted on yourself to show that are sorry for your sins.

The home

Although many hospitals were established in medieval England, the vast majority of sick people were cared for at home. It was expected that women would care for their relatives and dependents when needed. This care would have involved making the patient comfortable, preparing restorative foods and mixing herbal remedies.

Women would also be responsible for the garden, in which they were expected to grow various plants known for their healing properties, such as marigolds and clover.

Some historical sources hint that women in the home were well-respected for their healing skills. Letters written in 1464 between Lady Margaret Paston and her husband Sir John, when he was sick in London and she was at home worrying about him, show that neither of them trusted doctors and both would have been happier if he had been at home receiving treatment from her (see Source E).

Source E

An extract from a letter sent from Margaret Paston to her husband, John Paston, in 1464. The Pastons were wealthy landowners living in Norfolk. At the time that this letter was written, John Paston was staying in London.

For God's sake beware of any medicine that you get from any physicians in London. I shall never trust them because of what happened to your father and my uncle, whose souls God forgive.

Women likely had many more healing skills than just mixing herbal remedies and keeping the patient clean, warm and well-fed. There is some suggestion that they carried out minor surgeries and bleedings – however, records are very patchy. This might be because it was taken for granted that women cared for the sick, so nobody bothered to record it when it happened.

Exam-style question, Section B

'Hospital treatment in England in the period from 1250 to 1500 was very rare'.

How far do you agree? Explain your answer.

You may use the following information in your answer:

* charity hospitals
* care in the home.

You **must** also use information of your own. **20 marks**

Exam tip

This question gives an extra four marks for good spelling, grammar and punctuation, and the use of specialist terms. Take extra care over things like capital letters for key words.

Summary

* Religious treatments included prayer, fasting and pilgrimages.
* Supernatural treatments included saying spells or carrying amulets, although these were discouraged by the Church.
* There were a large number of treatments aimed at rebalancing the humours. This was normally done by eating a particular food, taking herbal remedies or by purging the body to remove bad humours, either by making the patient vomit or go to the toilet.
* Because there were no guaranteed treatments, medieval people were advised to avoid getting ill by living a healthy lifestyle and keeping clean.
* Physicians, apothecaries and barber surgeons all provided different treatments.
* Hospitals followed religious teachings. Patients were cared for and prayers were said, but they rarely received any medical treatment. However, most sick people were cared for in the home by a female family member.

Checkpoint

Strengthen

S1 What were the three different types of blood-letting?

S2 List the different ways people tried to prevent disease in medieval England.

S3 List the different sources of help sick people had in medieval England.

Challenge

C1 You need to show links between the treatments and remedies used in the Middle Ages, and the ideas people had about what caused disease. With this in mind, create a revision resource, matching what you learned about the causes of disease with what you have learned about treatments. This could take the form of a table, a poster or a 'pairs' game to play when you are revising.

C2 Add to your revision resource about treatments, linking the different sources of treatment to different beliefs about disease.

C3 Identify which different sources of treatment were available to different groups of people (for example: the rich, the poor, pregnant women, lepers).

If you do not feel confident answering any of these questions, discuss them with a partner or in a group.

1.3 Dealing with the Black Death, 1348–49

Learning outcomes

- Understand what the Black Death was and how it affected people in England during the years 1348-49.
- Understand the disputed causes, treatments and preventative measures used during the time of the Black Death.

In 1348, a new disease reached the shores of England. It had spread from the Far East along trade routes, arriving in Sicily in 1347, quickly spreading across the whole of Europe. The **Black Death**, as it eventually came to be known, was a new plague that was unfamiliar to the ordinary people of England, as well as English physicians. Within months, it had spread the length and breadth of England, killing thousands of people. It was absolutely devastating: it didn't matter if you were rich, poor, a city dweller or a country farmer – the plague did not discriminate. Those who caught it could expect to die within a matter of days.

Source A

This engraving from the 14th century shows somebody suffering from the Black Death.

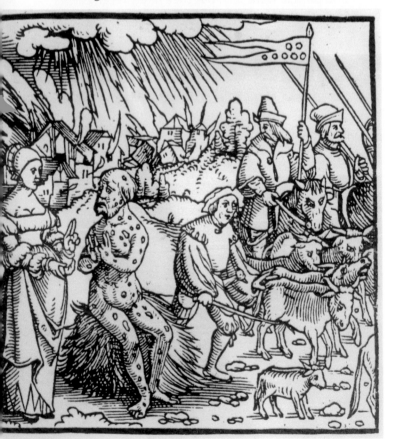

The disease still occurs every so often in modern times, but it is easily treated with antibiotics and patients usually make a full recovery, as long as it is caught in time. In the Middle Ages, treatments like this did not exist. People were completely unprepared, and they did not know how prevent and treat the 'scourge'*.

Key term

Scourge*

A person or thing that causes great suffering.

Source B

In this extract from a report on the Black Death written in 1347, Italian chronicler Marchione di Coppo Stefani describes how helpless people felt in the face of the epidemic (outbreak).

Neither physicians nor medicines were effective. Whether because these illnesses were previously unknown or because physicians had not previously studied them, there seemed to be no cure. There was such fear that nobody seemed to know what to do.

The Black Death

The Black Death was an outbreak of the bubonic plague. The bacteria were carried in the digestive system of fleas who arrived in England on rats carried by merchant ships. It was probably spread by flea bites, although some recent evidence suggests that it was also spread in the air. The main symptom was buboes, which was swelling in the armpit or groin, filled with pus.

Once caught, it was unlikely that you would survive the disease. It usually killed its victims in three to five days. At its height in London, 200 people were being buried every day. Contemporary accounts estimate that a third of the population of England died. Where the plague spread, it was common for more than half of a population of a town or city to die.

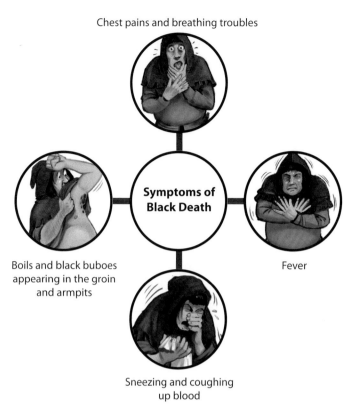

Figure 1.8 Symptoms of the Black Death.

The Black Death is the name given by Victorian historians to the particular outbreak of the plague in 1348. After this, the plague returned every 10–20 years, although it killed fewer people with each subsequent outbreak.

People applied the same knowledge they had about the causes of disease and illness to the plague. New treatments appeared and advice on how to avoid catching the disease spread quickly.

Causes of the Black Death

Religious and supernatural

Many believed that the Black Death was the result of God deserting mankind – that is, the Black Death was a punishment for the sin in the world.

In 1345, there was an unusual positioning of the planets Mars, Jupiter and Saturn, which astrologers interpreted as a sign that something wonderful or terrible was about to happen.

Natural causes

The main natural cause attributed to the Black Death was impure air. Breathing in this miasma caused corruption to the body's humours. People believed that this impure air may have originated from poisonous fumes released by an earthquake or a volcano.

Common beliefs

For the everyday people living in the cities and countryside, the spread of the Black Death was terrifying and they would have heard many conflicting ideas about what caused it. In Europe, many people blamed the Jewish population, but the Jews had been expelled from England in the 13th century, so this was not the case in England.

Treatments of the Black Death

Supernatural

The main recommendation to treat the Black Death was to confess your sins, and ask God for forgiveness through prayer. However, there was an air of inevitability about the disease: once caught, people believed it was clearly God's will; if it was his will that the patient should die, there was no cure that would work.

Natural

To begin with, physicians tried bleeding and purging – the same things they would usually do to correct a humoural imbalance. Unfortunately, that didn't work and, in fact, seemed to make people die more quickly.

As well as this, physicians recommended strong-smelling herbs like aloe and myrrh, which were believed to have cleansing properties. They often prescribed theriaca, as it was believed to work for lots of ailments. Lighting a fire and boiling vinegar could also drive off the bad air. Physicians or surgeons sometimes lanced the buboes – occasionally, people whose buboes burst survived.

Common beliefs

Everyday people were willing to try anything to survive the Black Death. They held strong Christian beliefs, and so would have gone to confession and prayed, as well as seeking traditional cures like bleeding. However, it quickly became clear that neither priests nor physicians were capable of curing the disease.

Activity ?

In groups of four, use the information above to create a television news report about the possible causes of the Black Death and what advice sufferers were given. One of you should play the part of a journalist, while the others take on the roles of priest, physician and an everyday person. Remember to give advice on both how to treat the disease and how to prevent it.

Apothecaries sold remedies and herbs were mixed in the home, based on old recipes, but they had uncertain and unpredictable results. Nobody came up with a cure that definitely worked in all cases.

The lack of medical knowledge about what **caused** the disease meant it was impossible to know how to **cure** it.

Preventing the Black Death

Supernatural means

The main advice given by priests was for people to:

- pray to God and fast
- go on a pilgrimage and make offerings to God
- show God how sorry you are by self-flagellation (whipping yourself). Large groups of flagellants wandered the streets of London, chanting and whipping themselves.

Natural means

Escaping the plague was the best advice for prevention. Guy de Chauliac, who was the physician to the Pope, advised people to: 'Go quickly, go far, and return slowly'. It was essential to escape the foul air to stay healthy.

If this kind of movement was impossible, people believed it was essential to carry a posy of flowers or fragrant herbs and hold it to your nose. This helped to avoid breathing in the miasma. Unlike the usual advice on preventing disease, people were advised to avoid bathing. It was believed that water would open the skin's pores to the corrupted air.

Common beliefs

One physician in Italy recommended doing joyful things, listening to cheerful music and avoiding anything sad as a protection against the disease. This is a clue as to just how desperate most physicians felt – they were willing to suggest anything to prevent their patients from catching the disease.

Much like the physicians, people did not know how to prevent the disease. However, they did stop visiting family members who had caught the plague – the common belief of the need to avoid those with the disease was so great that even their houses were avoided.

Key term

Quarantine*

Separating the sick from the healthy to stop the spread of a disease. Those who are sick are not allowed to leave the quarantined area.

Government action

Local authorities attempted to take action to prevent the plague from spreading. New quarantine* laws were put in place to try to stop people from moving around too much. People new to an area had to stay away from everybody else for 40 days, to ensure they were not carrying the disease. Authorities also started to quarantine houses where the plague had broken out. They considered banning preaching and religious processions, to stop large crowds of people gathering.

However, since the local government did not have a great deal of power at this time, they could not fully enforce these laws: rich people, for example, moved around quite freely and the Church continued to run as normal.

Because of the belief in bad air causing disease, the local authorities also stopped cleaning the streets. They believed that the foul stench of the rubbish and rotting bodies would drive off the miasma causing the plague.

Interpretation 1

Writer Sean Martin shares his views, and those of other historians, on the impact of the Black Death, in his book, *A Short History of Disease* (2015).

One immediate effect of the pandemic [an infectious disease spread across a large region] was the invention of quarantine. Historian GM Trevelyan argued that the Black Death was at least as important as the industrial revolution, while David Herlihy argued that the Black Death was "the great watershed", [an important turning point] without which there would have been no Renaissance, and with no Renaissance, no industrial revolution.

THINKING HISTORICALLY · Cause and Consequence

The language of causation

Study these words and phrases. They are useful in describing the role of causes and how they are related to each other and to events.

motivated	precondition	prevented	determined the timing	deepened the crisis	led to
exacerbated	allowed	triggered	impeded	catalyst	developed
underlying	created the potential	influenced	enabled	accelerated	sparked

1 Create a table with the following column headings: 'word', 'meaning', 'timing'. Write out each word or phrase in a separate row of the 'word' column.

2 Discuss the meaning of each word or phrase with a partner. For each word or phrase, write a short definition in the 'meaning' column.

3 Is each word or phrase more likely to describe a short-term, medium-term or long-term cause? In the 'timing' column, write 'short', 'medium' or 'long'.

4 Look at the following incomplete sentences. Write three versions of each sentence, using different words and phrases from the table to complete them. You can add extra words to make the sentences work. For each sentence, decide which version is the best.

   a   The power of the Church … the development of medical understanding.

   b   Following a regimen sanitatis … the prevention of disease.

   c   The lack of medical understanding … the spread of the Black Death.

5 You can also describe the importance of causes. Place the following words in order of importance. You should put words that suggest a cause is very important at the top, and words that suggest a cause is less important at the bottom of your list.

necessary	contributed to	added to	marginal	fundamental	influenced	supported	negligible

Summary

- Causes of the Black Death were thought to be supernatural – either as a result of alignment of the planets, a punishment from God – or caused by a miasma.
- Treatments included prayer, strong-smelling herbs and herbal remedies.
- To begin with, physicians tried bleeding and purging, but this made patients worse.
- Prevention was better than treatment: once you caught the Black Death, it was very likely that you would die.
- People tried to avoid catching the Black Death by avoiding infected family members or by leaving infected areas.
- Town authorities and other local governments tried to act by quarantining people.

Checkpoint

Strengthen

S1 Draw a flow diagram to show how the Black Death spread and the impact it had on Britain.

S2 Name four treatments people used to try to cure the Black Death.

S3 List reasons why the local authorities were not very successful in the methods they used to try to halt the spread of the Black Death.

Challenge

C1 How did people's beliefs about the causes of the Black Death, and ideas to prevent it, reflect general ideas about the causes of illness and disease from the period c1250–c1500? Create a 'Big picture, small detail' chart to match up ideas. An example is shown below.

Big Picture – general beliefs	Small detail – beliefs about the Black Death	Related treatment	Related prevention
God sent disease	The Black Death was a punishment for sin	Prayer, fasting	Prayer, fasting, pilgrimage, self-flagellation

How confident do you feel about your answers to these questions? Ask your teacher for some hints if you are stuck.

Recap: c1250–c1500: Medicine in medieval England

Recall quiz

1 Give two reasons why people believed God sent diseases.
2 Name two important classical medical thinkers.
3 What were the Four Humours?
4 What had to happen to the Four Humours to cause disease?
5 Name two other things people in the period c1250–c1500 believed caused disease.
6 What was theriaca?
7 What was the name for advice on how to maintain a healthy lifestyle?
8 What was the main job of the apothecary?
9 Roughly how many hospitals were there in England by 1500?
10 How many people died during the first outbreak of the plague in England?

Exam-style question, Section B

Explain why there was little change in the care provided by hospitals in the period c1250–c1500.

You may use the following information in your answer:

- ideas in the Church
- herbal remedies.

You **must** also use information of your own. **12 marks**

Exam tip

It's never too early to start timing your answers! A good rule of thumb is to allow yourself one and a half minutes per mark. You will need to both plan and write your answers in this time.

Activity

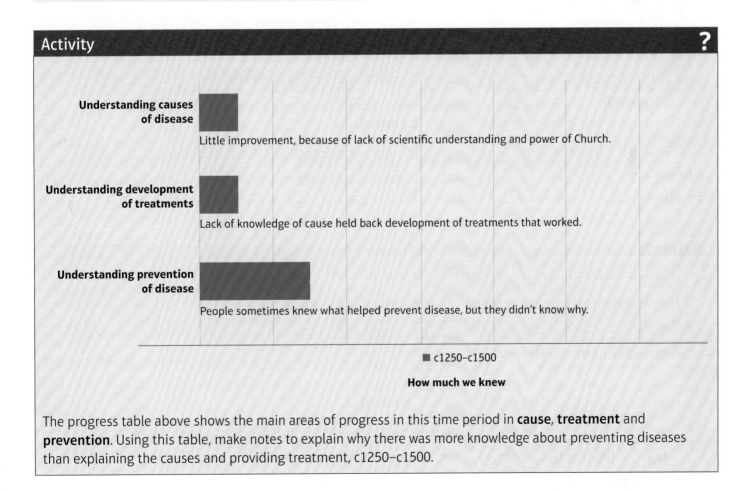

Understanding causes of disease — Little improvement, because of lack of scientific understanding and power of Church.

Understanding development of treatments — Lack of knowledge of cause held back development of treatments that worked.

Understanding prevention of disease — People sometimes knew what helped prevent disease, but they didn't know why.

■ c1250–c1500

How much we knew

The progress table above shows the main areas of progress in this time period in **cause**, **treatment** and **prevention**. Using this table, make notes to explain why there was more knowledge about preventing diseases than explaining the causes and providing treatment, c1250–c1500.

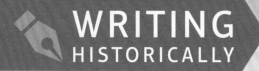

Writing historically: a clear response

Every response you write needs to be clearly written. To help you achieve this, you need to clearly signal that your response is relevant to the question you are answering.

Learning outcomes

By the end of this lesson, you will understand how to:

- use key noun phrases from the question to make sure you give a direct answer
- write short statements to express your ideas and opinions clearly, using a subject-verb construction.

Definitions

Noun: a word that names an object, idea, person, place, etc. (e.g. 'Black Death', 'disease', 'town').

Noun phrase: a phrase including a noun and any words that modify its meaning (e.g. 'the king of England').

Verb: words that describe actions ('Galen <u>developed</u> a theory'), incidents ('The disease <u>spread</u>') and situations ('Galen's theory <u>lasted</u> for centuries').

Subject-verb construction: A noun or noun phrase combined with a verb that tells you what the subject did or is doing.

How can I make sure I am answering the question?

Look at this exam-style question in which key nouns, noun phrases and verbs are highlighted:

> Explain why there was continuity in ideas about the cause of disease during the period c1250–c1500. **(12 marks)**

Now look at the first two sentences from two different responses to this question below.

Answer A

> Although the Church controlled medical learning, Galen's ideas on the cause of disease were accepted. Galen's ideas fitted in with the ideas of the Church.

Answer B

> Galen developed the Theory of Opposites. He also believed in the idea of a soul.

1. a. Which answer signals most clearly that it is going to answer the question?

   b. Write a sentence or two explaining your choice.

2. Now look at this exam-style question:

> Explain **one** way in which people's reactions to the plague were similar in the 14th and 17th centuries. **(4 marks)**

   a. Which are the key nouns, noun phrases and verbs in this question? Note them down.

   b. Write the first two sentences of your response to this question.

   c. In your opening sentences highlight any key words from the question. Have you used them all? If not, try rewriting your sentences, including all the words and phrases to signal that your response is answering the question clearly.

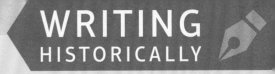
How can I clearly express my ideas?

One way to introduce your opinions and ideas clearly and briefly is by making short simple statements. Clear statements are often structured like this, using a subject-verb construction:

> *Galen developed the Four Humours into the Theory of Opposites. The Theory of Opposites and his ideas were in harmony with those of the Church.*

The verb tells you what happened.

The noun tells you who or what is the subject of the sentence.

This noun is the subject of the main verb. It tells you who or what the verb refers to.

3. Look again at Answer A's opening sentences:

> *Although the Church controlled medical learning, Galen's ideas on the cause of disease were accepted. Galen's ideas fitted in with the ideas of the Church.*

This short statement sentence expresses the writer's approach to the question clearly and briefly.

The writer could have written:

> *Because Galen's ideas on the cause of disease fitted in with the ideas of the Church, who controlled medical learning, they were accepted.*

or

> *Galen's ideas on the cause of disease were accepted as they fitted in with the ideas of the Church, even though the Church controlled medical learning.*

Which version do you prefer? Write a sentence or two explaining your choice.

4. a. Try rewriting the same information using different sentence structures to all the versions above.

   b. Can you make your version clearer or more concise than Answer A?

Improving an answer

Look at this exam question:

> Explain **one** way in which approaches to the treatment of disease were different in the 13th and 17th centuries. **(4 marks)**

Now look at one response to it:

> *Many people used herbal remedies. These were usually made with local plants and herbs such as mint and camomile. Recipes for these included theriaca, a popular remedy. More materials were available later due to increased overseas trading. New ingredients included nutmeg and cinnamon. There were also experiments with chemical cures, for example, the use of mercury to treat syphilis.*

5. Rewrite the response so that:

   a. it includes an opening sentence that focuses on key words and phrases from the question

   b. it includes a short statement sentence with a subject-verb construction to clearly introduce the approach to the question.

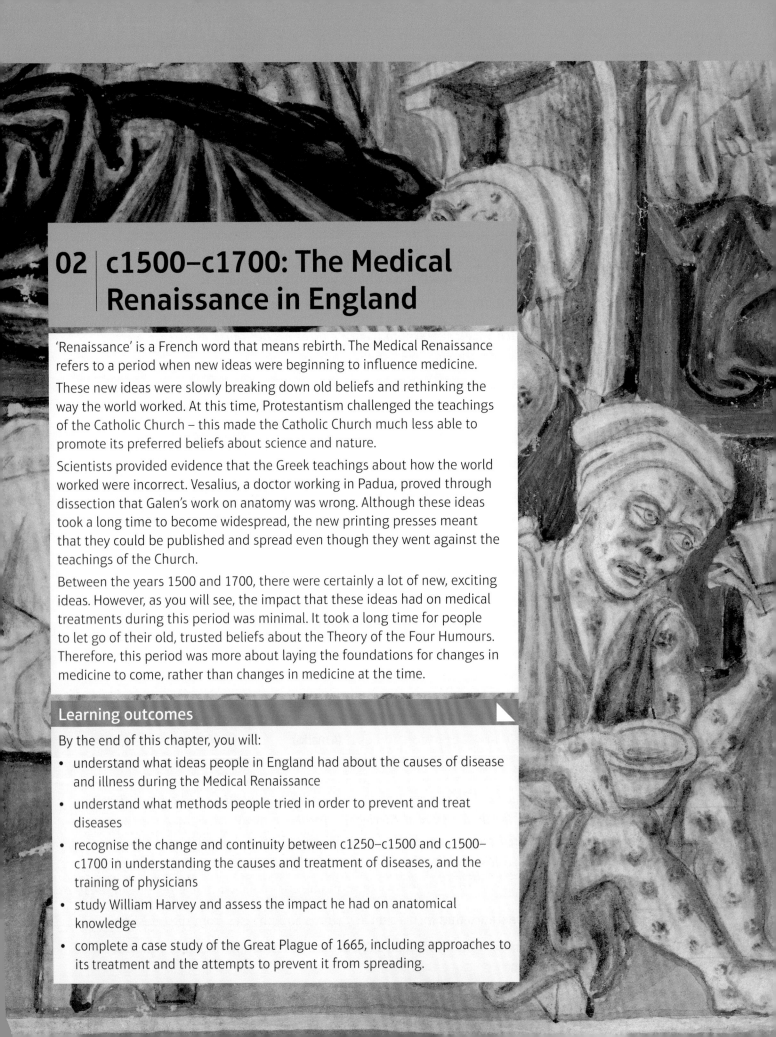

02 | c1500–c1700: The Medical Renaissance in England

'Renaissance' is a French word that means rebirth. The Medical Renaissance refers to a period when new ideas were beginning to influence medicine.

These new ideas were slowly breaking down old beliefs and rethinking the way the world worked. At this time, Protestantism challenged the teachings of the Catholic Church – this made the Catholic Church much less able to promote its preferred beliefs about science and nature.

Scientists provided evidence that the Greek teachings about how the world worked were incorrect. Vesalius, a doctor working in Padua, proved through dissection that Galen's work on anatomy was wrong. Although these ideas took a long time to become widespread, the new printing presses meant that they could be published and spread even though they went against the teachings of the Church.

Between the years 1500 and 1700, there were certainly a lot of new, exciting ideas. However, as you will see, the impact that these ideas had on medical treatments during this period was minimal. It took a long time for people to let go of their old, trusted beliefs about the Theory of the Four Humours. Therefore, this period was more about laying the foundations for changes in medicine to come, rather than changes in medicine at the time.

Learning outcomes

By the end of this chapter, you will:

- understand what ideas people in England had about the causes of disease and illness during the Medical Renaissance
- understand what methods people tried in order to prevent and treat diseases
- recognise the change and continuity between c1250–c1500 and c1500–c1700 in understanding the causes and treatment of diseases, and the training of physicians
- study William Harvey and assess the impact he had on anatomical knowledge
- complete a case study of the Great Plague of 1665, including approaches to its treatment and the attempts to prevent it from spreading.

2.1 Ideas about the cause of disease and illness

• Understand the different ideas about the causes of disease that changed and stayed the same, c1500–c1700.

Ideas about disease and illness: change and continuity

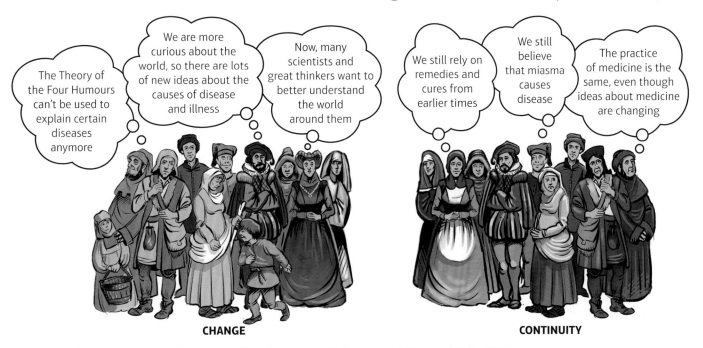

Figure 2.1 Change and continuity surrounding the causes of disease and illness, c1500–c1700.

People who fell ill during the period 1500 to 1700 were likely to believe the same things about the cause of their illness as their medieval ancestors. Very little really changed in the practice of medicine during this period.

However, all across Europe, enormous shifts were taking place in other areas of daily life. Beautiful art was being created in new styles and with new techniques; beliefs were changing, with new forms of Christianity and a more secular* society developing; and understanding of the surrounding world was increasing with scientific discoveries.

Key word

Secular*

Not religious or in any way connected with spiritual beliefs.

Because of these changes, medical knowledge grew with the changing attitudes of ordinary people. The general population of Europe wanted better answers to the questions about what caused disease. Epidemics of the plague and other killer diseases, such as smallpox, the Great Pox (syphilis) and sweating sickness, could not be easily explained by the Theory of the Four Humours. They affected everybody in the same way and were not cured by traditional humoural treatments, like blood-letting and purging.

There was still a widespread belief in miasmata as a cause of humoural imbalance and disease. A miasma could be the product of rotten vegetables, decaying bodies of humans or animals, excrement or any swampy, smelly, dirty place. However, even this did not provide a satisfactory explanation for the spread of diseases when people took such care to avoid miasma.

Some people came up with new ideas about the causes of disease and illness. They included new ideas based on alchemy* and new discoveries about the body. Some of these new ideas are listed in the table below, together with the name of the scientist or doctor who discovered them.

> **Key word**
>
> **Alchemy***
>
> This was an early form of chemistry. Alchemists tried to turn one material into another: mostly, they were trying to discover a way of making gold.

New ideas and discoveries in the period c1500–c1700

New ideas about disease and illness	Influential individual
In the 16th century, the Theory of the Four Humours was rejected by some radical physicians. Disease was seen as something separate from the body, which needed to be attacked. New chemical treatments started to appear, influenced by the increasing popularity of alchemy.	Paracelsus, a Swiss scientist and medical professor.
In 1546, a new text called *On Contagion* theorised that disease was caused by seeds spread in the air.	Girolamo Fracastoro, an Italian physician.
In 1628, a new theory was published in Britain, which suggested that blood circulated around the body instead of being made in the liver, as taught by Galen.	William Harvey, an English scientist
A better understanding of the digestive system developed. This meant that people gradually stopped believing disease was caused by eating the wrong things. Urine was no longer seen as an accurate way of diagnosing illness.	Jan Baptiste van Helmont, a Flemish physician.
New microscopes were being developed, which allowed for much clearer magnification. A new book, *Micrographia*, published in 1665, showed many detailed images, including a close-up drawing of a flea, copied from a magnified image.	Robert Hooke, an English scientist and head of experiments at the Royal Society.
In 1676, the medical textbook *Observationes Medicae* was published. This theorised that illness was caused by external factors, rather than the four humours.	Thomas Sydenham, an English physician. (see page 44)
By 1683, more powerful microscopes had been developed to allow for the observation of tiny 'animalcules' or little animals in plaque scraped from between the teeth. The images were not very clear, but they were visible. This was the first recorded observation of bacteria.	Antony van Leeuwenhoek, a Dutch scientist (see page 46).

So, due to all these new discoveries and ideas, by c1700:

- the Theory of the Four Humours had been discredited – however, it was still being followed by the general population of Britain
- other ideas about causes of disease had been discovered (for example, 'animalcules').

Even though some of these ideas were very close to what we now know as the truth, they had very little impact at the time. This was due to several reasons.

A better understanding of human anatomy (the makeup of the body) was developing all the time. However, there was no point studying correct drawings of the internal organs when it was impossible to diagnose or treat internal problems on a living patient.

Also, the lack of quality medical instruments, such as microscopes, prevented any rapid change in people's beliefs about the causes of disease. The new theories might have been very convincing, but without scientific proof they were just that – theories.

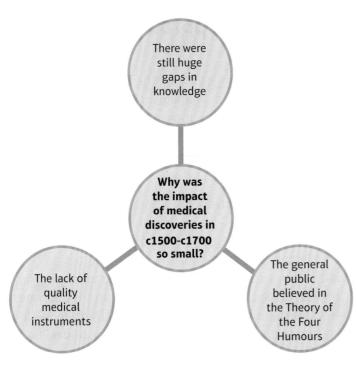

Figure 2.2 Why was the impact of scientific discoveries up to 1700 so small?

Because the general public believed in the Theory of the Four Humours, most physicians stuck to the old methods. They were in the business of healing the sick, not coming up with better methods of doing it. Even those who did look for new ideas still needed to work, and patients did not want to pay physicians to experiment on them.

Changing ideas

The key point to note here is that, while the **practice** of medicine did not change much at this time, **ideas** were starting to change. Scientists like Galileo and Copernicus were challenging the authority of the Church in other areas of scientific understanding. This encouraged medical scientists to start looking beyond the works of Galen and Hippocrates. By the end of the 17th century, doctors and scientists had lots of new ideas about the causes of illness and disease – it just wasn't applied to everyday medical practice.

Below is a chart that shows how ideas about the causes of disease and illness changed during the Medical Renaissance.

Ideas that changed a lot	Ideas that changed a little	Ideas that stayed the same
The Theory of the Four Humours. Very few physicians believed this by the end of the 17th century, though it was still used when diagnosing disease, because patients understood it.	**The use of medical books.** Physicians carried out more observations of their patients. However, they still relied on texts for looking up symptoms.	**Miasmata.** The idea that disease was spread by bad smells and evil fumes was constant throughout this period – and even became more widespread during epidemics.
The human body. There was a much better understanding of anatomy.	**The influence of the Church.** Most people now recognised that God did not send disease. However, in times of epidemics, such as during the Great Plague, religious causes were still considered.	
Diagnosis using urine. Physicians now understood that urine was not directly related to a person's health.	**Supernatural**. Although astrology was much less popular from 1500, in times of epidemics people still wore charms to ward off the disease.	

Activity ?

Draw two columns and label the first one 'Old ideas', and the second one 'New ideas'. Using the information in this chapter, and things you have already learned in Chapter 1, make brief notes on ideas about the causes of illness and disease in the years c1500–c1700 that were the same as c1250–c1500, and the ideas that were different.

Exam-style question, Section B

Explain **one** way in which ideas about the cause of disease and illness were similar in the 14th and 17th centuries.
4 marks

Exam tip

This answer should not be very long, but it does need to have specific information for each time period. Try to make a general point that covers both time periods – for example, the idea of miasmata – and then give a specific example for each time period.

Source A

A drawing of Thomas Sydenham, by an unknown artist, after his death.

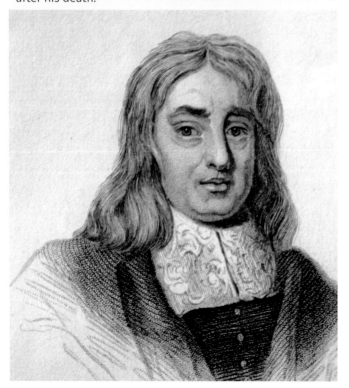

A scientific approach to diagnosis

One of the key changes during the Renaissance was the rise of **humanism**. Humanism was characterised by a love of learning, a new interest in classical scholars and the belief that human beings could make up their own minds when it came to discovering the truth of the world around them.

Humanism also represented a break with some of the old medieval traditions. Humanists rejected the Christian view that God was responsible for everything that happened, but they hadn't yet figured out an alternative explanation. People returned to the original texts of ancient scholars such as Galen and Hippocrates. New translations of the works of Hippocrates and Galen started to appear. During the 16th century, 590 editions of Galen's writings were published.

During the 17th century, more experimentation began to take place in the field of medicine. This, in part, was because the Church had less authority in everyday life. Proof that Galen had been wrong about the human anatomy was becoming more widespread, thanks to the work of Vesalius (see pages 52–55). New ideas were starting to gain more support, although it would be a long time before this had an impact on everyday medical treatment.

Thomas Sydenham

Thomas Sydenham was nicknamed 'the English Hippocrates'. He was a well-respected doctor in London in the 1660s and 1670s. The Theory of the Four Humours was still being used at this time, but it was starting to lose popularity. Sydenham's work was very important in moving medicine in Britain away from the classical ideas of Galen and Hippocrates, and into the new era.

Sydenham refused to rely on medical books when diagnosing a patient's illness. Instead, he made a point of closely observing the symptoms and treating the disease causing them. This was a change from the medieval method of treating each of the symptoms separately, instead of seeing them all as side effects of one cause.

Source B

Thomas Sydenham published his theories about disease and his observations of various epidemics in a book called *Observationes Medicae* in 1676. In this extract from the introduction, he explains that doctors should devote as much time to identifying different types of disease as botanists spend identifying different types of plant.

In the first place, it is necessary that all diseases be reduced to definite and certain species, and that, with the same care which we see exhibited by botanists [specialists in the scientific study of plants]; since it happens, at present, that many diseases... are... different in their natures, and require a different medical treatment. We should have known the cures of many diseases before this time if physicians, whilst with all due good-will they communicated their experiments and observations, had not been deceived in their disease, and had not mistaken one species for another.

One of Sydenham's most controversial ideas was that diseases were like plants and animals, in that they could be organised into different groups. According to the Theory of the Four Humours, a patient's disease was personal to them: it was caused by any number of individual factors, including the weather, diet and the patient's particular balance of humours, which differed from person to person. This meant that treatments also varied from person to person.

Sydenham did not believe this. He encouraged his students to observe their patients, note down their symptoms in detailed descriptions and then look for remedies to tackle the disease. He theorised that the nature of the patient had little to do with the disease.

This was a very modern idea and laid the foundations for a more scientific approach to medicine from the 18th century onwards. Sydenham was not able to isolate and identify the various microorganisms that caused the diseases that he was observing. However, he was able to identify that measles and scarlet fever were separate diseases.

Extend your knowledge

Thomas Sydenham's new treatments

Thomas Sydenham developed a number of new treatments to tackle the diseases he identified. Instead of using the popular 'sweating' method for treating smallpox, he prescribed airy bedrooms, light blankets and cold drinks. He also popularised the use of cinchona bark from Peru to treat malaria. Cinchona contains quinine which is still used to treat malaria today.

Activities

1 List the effects humanism had on medicine during the Medical Renaissance.

2 Draw a stick figure to represent Thomas Sydenham. Add thought bubbles to detail his ideas about medicine.

3 Investigating the causes of disease and isolating different types was very important in the fight against disease. Imagine you are a doctor in the 17th century. Write a proposal or letter addressing other doctors, explaining how you think Sydenham's ideas could be used to improve medical treatments.

Improved communications

One of the changes across Europe during the Medical Renaissance was the improvement in literacy: more people than ever before were able to read and write. This meant new ideas could spread further and more quickly.

The influence of the printing press

In around 1440, Johannes Gutenberg, a German goldsmith, created the world's first printing press*. It didn't take long for the popularity of his new invention to grow: by 1500, there were hundreds of presses in Europe.

Key term

Printing press*

A machine for printing text or pictures. It had movable letters so that many copies of the same text could be printed.

The new printing press enabled information to be spread accurately and quickly. Text no longer had to be copied by hand, meaning there were fewer inconsistencies in the same version of a text. It also meant that scientists could publish their work and share it across Europe much faster than when the work had to be copied by hand.

The printing press also took book copying out of the hands of the Church. This meant that a much wider variety of subjects were written about, whereas, before this time, most books were about religious topics. The Church was no longer able to prevent ideas they disapproved of being published. For example, physicians could now publish works criticising Galen.

The work of the Royal Society

The desire to explain the world in secular terms led to a big increase in the number of experiments being carried out. Scientists wanted to talk to each other about their new discoveries and share new ideas. This led to the founding of the **Royal Society**.

The Royal Society met for the first time at Gresham College in London, in 1660. Its aim was to promote and carry out experiments to further the understanding of science. They also heavily promoted the sharing of scientific knowledge and encouraged argument over new theories and ideas. In 1662, the society received its royal charter* from Charles II, who had a keen interest in science.

Key term

Royal charter*

A document from the monarch, granting a right or power to a particular person or group. A Royal Charter shows that the monarch is supportive of a particular project.

The support of the king gave the Royal Society credibility: if the king approved of and supported them, clearly they were doing something right. It also raised their profile. More people sent their work in to be published, or were willing to donate money supporting the scientific work of the Royal Society.

Extend your knowledge

The Royal Society

The motto of the Royal Society was '*Nullius in verba*'. This means 'Take nobody's word for it'. It shows that at the heart of the Royal Society was a desire to find new scientific discoveries through experimenting and evidence.

In 1665, the Society began publishing their scientific journal, called *Philosophical Transactions*. It was the world's first scientific journal, and it continues to be published today, celebrating its 350th anniversary in 2015.

Source C

This picture of 'animalcules' was drawn to go with a letter Antony van Leeuwenhoek had published in *Philosophical Transactions* in 1702. The letter was titled 'Concerning green weeds growing in water, and some animalcula growing about them'.

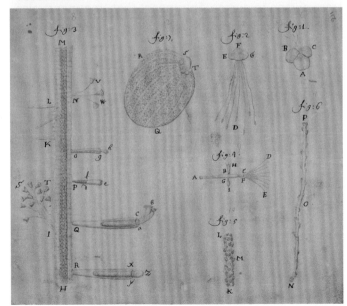

When it was first published, the journal consisted of letters, book reviews and summaries of experiments and observations carried out by European scientists. *Philosophical Transactions* provided a vitally important platform from which scientists could share their work, and therefore contributed a great deal to the spread of medical ideas. For example, they published several letters from Leeuwenhoek, in which he described his observations of 'animalcules'.

The Royal Society offered funding for translations of European scientific texts. It encouraged its members to write their reports in English instead of Latin, and in straightforward language, to make it accessible for everyone. It also requested that members provide a copy of any of their submissions, which would be put into a reference library and made available for anybody to study.

The Royal Society made it possible for physicians and scientists to access and study each others' research. It was therefore very important in the development of new medical ideas.

When Leeuwenhoek's work (see Source C) was received by the Royal Society, they gave it to their microscope enthusiast, Robert Hooke. Hooke used his own microscope to confirm what Leeuwenhoek had seen. Because it was published in *Philosophical Transactions*, news of the new discovery spread quickly and widely.

THINKING HISTORICALLY Change and continuity (2a)

Distinguishing between change and continuity

Change is happening all the time. Every day, things change slightly in lots of different ways. For example, ten more people in the country might be unemployed today compared to yesterday, or mobile phone batteries might have become 1% more powerful. Most of these changes are small, and not important enough to be called 'change' by historians.

Study the following events that demonstrate changes in understanding the causes of disease.

1526 Paracelsus theorised that disease was caused by problems with chemicals inside the body

1546 Fracastoro wrote a text called *On Contagion*, suggesting that disease was caused by seeds that spread in the air

1628 Harvey proved that blood circulates around the body

1648 Van Helmont claimed that digestion happened because of stomach acid, rather than anything to do with the Four Humours

1665 Hooke developed a more powerful microscope and published a book of images from his observations

1676 Thomas Sydenham published *Observationes Medicae*, theorising that diseases were separate from the patient, rather than being caused by something the patient did

1683 Leeuwenhoek developed a microscope and observed 'animalcules', or 'little animals'

1 Using only three events in the list, write a paragraph explaining how understanding about the causes of disease changed during this period. Think carefully about which events you include.

A period of 'continuity' is a period of time when very little (if anything) changes.

2 Can you identify any periods of continuity in the timeline when looking at ideas about the causes of disease?

3 If you identified a period of continuity, write down:

   a what it was that stayed the same over that period

   b what, if anything, changed.

4 Write your own definitions of 'change' and 'continuity'.

Exam-style question, Section B

Explain why there were changes in the way ideas about the causes of disease and illness were communicated in the period c1500–c1700.

You may use the following in your answer:

- the printing press
- the Royal Society.

You **must** also use information of your own. **12 marks**

Exam tip

Make sure that you fully explain your points by using the **P**oint, **E**xample, **E**xplain, or **PEE** method. State your argument, then add some examples from your own knowledge to back it up. Finish off by explaining how that evidence relates to the question.

Summary

- There was very little change in medical practice. Methods of diagnosing illness remained similar to medieval times.
- Lots of new ideas about the causes of disease and illness started to appear, but they were slow to have an impact on patients.
- By the end of the 17th century, most doctors no longer believed that humoural imbalance caused disease, although they still referred to the Theory of the Four Humours when diagnosing disease.
- There was a new fashion for careful observation and believing what you saw over what you read. Thomas Sydenham was important in promoting this method in England.
- The invention of the printing press made it easier for physicians to share their work.
- From the middle of the 17th century onwards, the Royal Society promoted scientific experimentation, funded research and provided a hub for sharing ideas and discoveries.

Checkpoint

Strengthen

S1 What new ideas about the causes of disease and illness started to appear at this time?

S2 What was humanism and how did it affect ideas about the causes of illness and disease?

S3 Who was Thomas Sydenham and what new ideas did he have?

S4 How did the Royal Society encourage the development of medical ideas?

Challenge

C1 How important was new technology in enabling the development of new ideas about the causes of disease and illness?

C2 How far did individuals and institutions in the 17th century help lead to new discoveries?

If you are not confident about any of these questions, form a group with other students, discuss the answers and then record your conclusions. Your teacher can give you some hints.

2.2 Approaches to prevention and treatment

Treatment: change and continuity

Since belief in humoural imbalances persisted through to the end of the 17th century and beyond, the old treatments, which were aimed at rebalancing humours, continued as well. Bleeding, purging and sweating were all popular ways of removing too much of a particular humour.

A new popular theory in this period was the idea of **transference** – which meant that an illness or a disease could be transferred to something else. For example, people believed that if you rubbed an object on an ailment (such as a boil), the disease would transfer from you to the object. There was also a popular theory that you could get rid of warts by rubbing them with an onion – through transference, the warts would 'transfer' to the vegetable!

Extend your knowledge

Transference

Some patients with a fever used to sleep with a sheep in the bedroom, hoping that their fever would transfer to the animal.

Herbal remedies continued to be popular, although their use changed slightly. In c1500–c1700, often remedies were chosen because of their colour or shape. For example, yellow herbs, such as radish and saffron, were used to treat jaundice (which turns the skin yellow). Smallpox, which had a red rash as one of the symptoms, was treated with the 'red cure' – drinking red wine, eating red foods and wearing red clothes.

Since this was the age of exploration, new herbal remedies started to appear from other countries. New plants started to appear from the New World*.

Source A

In 1652, Nicholas Culpeper published his book *The English Physitian: Or An Astrologo-Physicial Discourse of the Vulgar Herbs of This Nation*. Culpeper brought together all the information from the medieval *Materia Medica* and wrote it in English to make it available for everybody.

Vervain is hot and dry, opening obstructions, cleansing and healing. It helps the yellow jaundice, the dropsy and the gout; it kills and expels worms in the belly, and causes a good colour in the face and body, strengthens as well as corrects the diseases of the stomach, liver and spleen; helps the cough, wheezings and shortness of breath, and all the defects of the veins and bladder, expelling the gravel and stone.

Some physicians believed that within each country were herbal remedies which would cure the diseases that came from that country: the appearance of new remedies opened up a huge number of new possibilities for treatments and cures.

New remedies that started to appear included sarsaparilla from the New World, used to treat the Great Pox, and ipecacuanha from Brazil, later known just as ipecac, which was effective as a cure for dysentery*. Thomas Sydenham popularised the use of cinchona bark, from Peru, in treating malaria. This was an effective remedy as long as patients continued to take it for some time after it seemed as though the disease had gone. Physicians also tested other new arrivals like tea, coffee, nutmeg, cinnamon and even tobacco to see if they had any impact on diseases.

Key words

New World*

North and South America. Europeans were only aware of their existence from 1492.

Dysentery*

A stomach bug that causes severe diarrhoea.

Chemical cures

The growth of alchemy, which laid the foundations for the modern science of chemistry, had an impact on medical treatments. People began to look for chemical cures for diseases instead of relying on herbs and blood-letting. This new science was known as **iatrochemistry**, or **medical chemistry**, and it was extremely popular in the 17th century.

Inspired by Paracelsus, the scientist who experimented with chemical treatments, medical chemists experimented with metals as cures for common ailments. The *Pharmacopoeia Londinensis*, published by the College of Physicians in 1618 as a manual of remedies, included a chapter on salts, metals and minerals. Among its 2,140 remedies were 122 different chemical preparations, including mercury and antimony. In small doses, antimony promotes sweating, which cools the body down. This fitted in with the idea of purging the body of disease. Patients would leave wine in an antimony cup overnight and drink the contents in the morning. In larger doses, antimony was used to encourage vomiting – another type of purge. Although it is poisonous in its pure form, a compound of it, known as antimony potassium tartrate, was said to have cured Louis XIV of France of typhoid fever in 1657, and became wildly popular afterwards.

Source B

This woodcut, published in a French medical textbook by Hannibal Barlet in 1657, shows a patient vomiting after being given antimony as a purge.

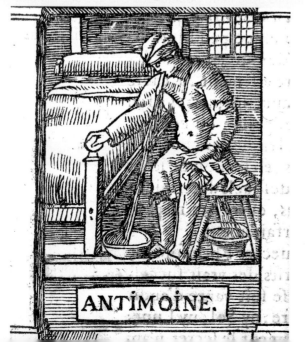

ANTIMOINE.

Prevention: change and continuity

Preventing disease was still considered to be the best way to avoid dying from it: since treatments had not moved on from medieval times, there was still no certainty that a person would recover. The only sure way to avoid dying from a disease, therefore, was not catching one at all.

People believed you could avoid disease by practising moderation in all things, as well as avoiding draughts, exhaustion, rich and fatty foods, too much strong alcohol and being too lazy. Condition at birth was also important – being born small or weak might be used to explain death from an illness in adulthood. This idea of a person's 'constitution' was related to the medieval idea of a person's humours and personality being influenced by the season in which they were born.

Cleanliness was also still important – both the home and the body needed to be kept clean and free from bad smells. However, bathing had become a lot less fashionable in England since the arrival of syphilis.

Syphilis had spread so quickly among people who regularly visited the stewes, or bathhouses, in London that Henry VIII had been forced to close them down in the early 16th century. The spread of syphilis at these places was probably, in part, due to the fact that many bathhouses were also brothels. However, the link between syphilis and bathhouses was not easily forgotten, and it was thought that bathing led to people catching the disease. People in the 16th and 17th centuries were far more likely to keep themselves clean by rubbing themselves down with linen and changing their clothes regularly than by going to public baths.

People continued to try to avoid catching diseases by practising **regimen sanitatis**. However, by the end of the 17th century, avoidance methods were as much about changing your surroundings (moving away from an area with a disease) as they were about looking after yourself. The idea that certain weather conditions, or the surrounding atmosphere, spread disease was becoming more popular. New instruments like **barometers** and **thermometers** were used to measure and record weather conditions over a long period of time, to see if there was a link between the weather and outbreaks of disease.

More steps were also taken to remove miasmata from the air. Homeowners in English towns were fined for not cleaning the street outside their house. Projects were set up to drain swamps and bogs. Removing sewage and picking up rubbish from the streets was a punishment given to minor criminals.

Activities

1 There are lots of unusual new words in this chapter, like iatrochemistry. Create a glossary for at least five of them. Write the words and their definition. You could also do this on flash cards.

2 Make a list of all the new treatments described in this chapter that appeared between 1500 and 1700. How many of them are newer versions of old treatments and how many of them are completely new?

3 What influences encouraged people to try new treatments? Work through the text above, identifying different things that changed medical treatment and matching them to your list from the first activity. For example, you might label sarsaparilla and ipecacuanha 'Influenced by exploration of the New World'.

Exam-style question, Section B

Explain **one** way in which ideas about the treatment of disease were different in the 17th century from ideas in the 13th century.   **4 marks**

Exam tip

The difference between half marks and full marks on this question is how precise your knowledge is. Make sure you give a fact that relates to each time period.

Preventing disease: things that were the same (continuity)	Preventing disease: things that were different (change)
People still believed that there were many factors that could prevent disease, including superstitions and prayer…	…but people also started to believe that other things could help avoid disease, such as practising moderation and your condition at birth.
Cleanliness was still very important…	…but bathing had become a lot less fashionable in England since the arrival of syphilis. People now kept clean by changing their clothes more often.
People continued to practise regimen sanitatis…	…but, by the end of the 17th century, people also began to think that disease was also related to other factors (for example, the weather).
Miasma was still believed in…	…but more steps were now taken to remove miasma from the air (for example, removing sewage and picking up rubbish from the streets).

Medical care: change and continuity

The same range of professionals offered treatment from c1500–c1700 as in the period c1250–c1500: trained physicians, apothecaries and surgeons. However, there were some changes.

Apothecaries and surgeons

Apothecaries continued to mix remedies and surgeons continued to carry out simple operations during the Medical Renaissance. In the period c1250–c1500, apothecaries were organised into **guild systems**. This meant that men would carry out an apprenticeship, and then spend several years practising as a journeyman* under the supervision of a master, before becoming a master surgeon or apothecary himself.

Key term

Journeyman*

An experienced member of a profession who was not yet experienced enough to have his own business. Journeymen usually worked for a master until they had enough expertise to start their own business.

Education for both types of medical professional increased considerably between 1500 and 1700. With wars being fought with new technology, new wounds on the battlefield meant that more surgery was necessary, while the introduction of iatrochemistry introduced new ingredients into the stores of apothecaries. Both surgeons and apothecaries had to possess licences to be able to practice their trade. Surgeons and apothecaries continued to provide services to those unable to afford physicians.

Physicians

Physicians continued to be trained at universities in the period c1500–c1700. Training courses changed very little during this period: there were some new ideas emerging, but, as with diagnosis and treatment, they were slow to take effect.

Although new subjects were introduced into the medical curriculum, like iatrochemistry and anatomy, most learning was still from books and not from practical experience. Lectures were dictated in Latin. However, as new ideas about human anatomy and iatrochemistry started to be shared, doctors were inspired to challenge the old teachings and investigate for themselves. This was particularly the case in the 17th century, when the Hippocratic focus on observation became more popular.

However, there was still very little practical, hands-on training. Dissection, which had once been banned by the Church, was legalised due to the decline in the power of the Church, but it was still very difficult to get a supply of fresh corpses to dissect. Very few universities had an anatomy theatre, because most of them didn't think it was necessary to train a physician in anatomy – after all, he would only need it if he was supervising a lowly surgeon.

Luckily, trainee doctors had much better access to medical textbooks and there were a wider variety of these books than ever before. The newly-invented printing press made books easier to find and a lot cheaper. Protestantism rejected highly-decorated churches, so many artists found themselves with hours to spare and in need of work. This meant that they were available to create detailed drawings for these new medical textbooks. For medical students who couldn't afford a whole book, individual copies of pictures were available. These were known as **fugitive sheets**.

Andreas Vesalius

The most famous anatomist of this period was Andreas Vesalius. He studied medicine in Paris in 1533. Paris was a centre for the new humanist ideas about medicine. From there he went to Padua, which had a very famous university, where he became a lecturer in surgery. Vesalius had a deep interest in the human body and was keen to share his discoveries with the rest of the world.

His first publication in 1537, *Six Anatomical Tables*, showed the different parts of the human body, labelled in Latin, Greek, Hebrew and Arabic. Three of the six drawings showed a human skeleton, which Vesalius himself had assembled. He used the publication in his lectures: they were very popular with his students and colleagues.

Source C

A fugitive sheet printed in 1566 as an addition to an anatomical book by Valverde, a Spanish doctor.

Fugitive sheets were prints of anatomical drawings that were made for medical students. They usually featured layers of paper that could be lifted to show the body during various stages of dissection.

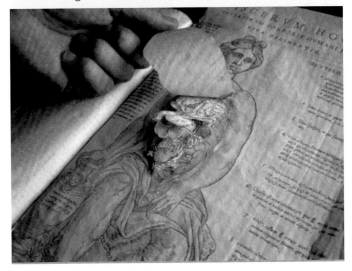

Six years later, in 1543, Vesalius published the book for which he is most famous: *De Humani Corporis Fabrica*, or *On the Fabric of the Human Body*. He had been able to carry out a large number of dissections, thanks to a local magistrate who allowed him to use the bodies of executed criminals.

Vesalius noted that Galen had made some errors in his original theory on the human body. He put this down to the fact that Galen dissected animals instead of people. In all, Vesalius found around 300 mistakes in Galen's original work on anatomy. These included:

- the human lower jaw was in one part, not two
- the vena cava (the main vein leading out of the heart) did not lead to the liver
- men did not have one fewer pair of ribs than women
- the human liver did not have five separate lobes
- the human breastbone was in three parts, not seven.

As well as correcting these mistakes, Vesalius encouraged other doctors to base their work on dissection rather than believing old books. He wrote that it was vital that anatomy professors carry out

Source D

This illustration is from Vesalius's book, *On the Fabric of the Human Body*. It is titled *'Fourth Muscle Dissection'*. There are 14 muscle dissection pictures in total: eight drawn from the front and six drawn from the back. In each one, Vesalius has stripped back another layer of muscle from the human body to reveal what is underneath. The final picture in each sequence shows the body supported by walls or blocks, as the substance of the limbs is cut away.

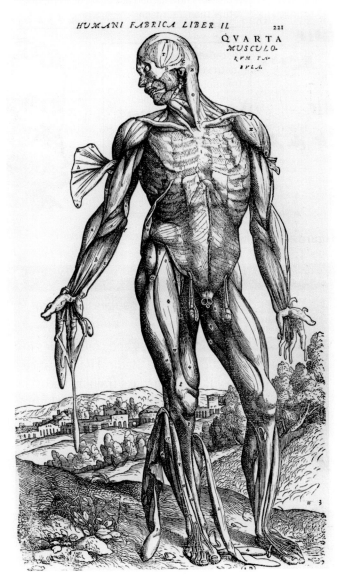

dissections for themselves, and claimed that this was really important if further advances in medical knowledge were to be made. Because of this, Vesalius laid the foundation for others to investigate the anatomy of the human body in more detail.

Vesalius's book was richly illustrated with incredibly detailed drawings of the human body in various stages of dissection. By including so many pictures, Vesalius hoped to present the ideal version of the human body, to which other dissected corpses could be compared.

It was not difficult to find artists willing to do this work: Renaissance artists were keen to study anatomy so that they could paint the human form more accurately and secure more work.

Made the study of anatomy not only acceptable, but fashionable. Anatomy became a central part of the study of medicine. Doctors and medical professors now carried out dissections themselves, rather than a surgeon.

His work was heavily copied, and even plagiarised. Versions of the drawings from the *Fabrica* appeared in other medical texts and as fugitive sheets.

He caused a huge controversy. A lot of traditional physicians were angry that he had criticised Galen. They said that the differences Vesalius had found were down to the fact that there had been changes in the human body since the time of Galen.

Inspired other anatomists, some of whom went on to correct his own mistakes in *Fabrica*.

He was a trail blazer. After he died, Fabricius discovered valves in human veins. Fabricius shared this work with his students at Padua – one of whom was William Harvey, who went on to discover the circulation of the blood.

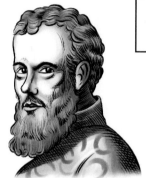

Vesalius

Figure 2.3 The impact of Vesalius.

Activities ?

1 Which individuals impacted changes in medical care between 1500 and 1700?

2 Draw a table to show changes and continuities in medical training during the 'Medical Renaissance'. How much do you think medical training had changed by 1700 – a little bit, some or a lot? Explain why you think this.

3 Vesalius is a key individual in the development of anatomy. Can you explain why he had an impact?

Extend your knowledge

Andreas Vesalius

As a humanist, Vesalius did not reject the ideas of Galen outright. There is evidence to suggest that he felt he was just completing a body of work begun by the ancient scholars. The title page to his book *Fabrica* shows Vesalius dissecting a woman while Galen, Hippocrates and Aristotle look on (see Source E). Vesalius hoped that, by correcting the errors in Galen's work on anatomy, more people would begin to use the ancient texts.

Exam-style question, Section B

'Individuals had the biggest impact on medical training in the 16th and 17th centuries'.

How far do you agree? Explain your answer.

You may use the following information in your answer:

- Vesalius
- the printing press.

You **must** also use some information of your own.

16 marks

Exam tip

This question asks you to consider the impact of one factor on medical training – individuals. Your counter-argument should focus on the impact of other factors. The bullet point is giving you a hint here by mentioning the printing press, a technological impact.

Source E

This is the first page of *Fabrica*. In it, Vesalius is dissecting a body whilst surrounded by a large crowd of people, including Galen. When his book was published, Vesalius dedicated it to the Holy Roman Emperor, Charles V, and presented him with a hand-coloured copy. By doing this he hoped that his book would be more respected by the wider medical community. Charles V must have liked what he saw, because he later offered Vesalius the job of personal physician!

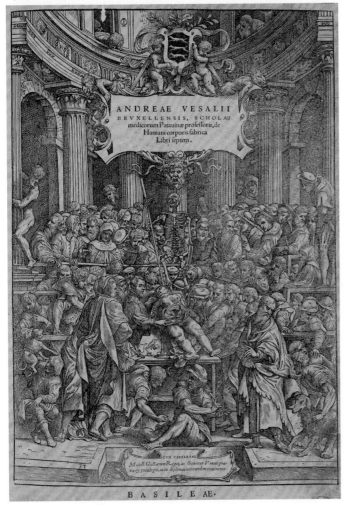

Caring for the sick: change and continuity

Hospitals

Some changes had begun to take place in English hospitals by the early 16th century. Whereas before, travellers, pilgrims, the elderly, and a few sick people would have attended hospitals for food, shelter and prayer, this had begun to change. Patient records suggest that many people went to hospital with wounds and curable diseases such as fevers and skin conditions. They didn't spend very long in the hospital before being discharged: this suggests that they got better.

A patient in a 16th-century hospital could expect:

- a good diet – the restorative effects of food were still important, as many people didn't have access to a lot of food that was good for them
- a visit from a physician – hospitals had contracts with doctors, who would visit the patients sometimes as often as twice a day, to observe the symptoms and prescribe treatments
- medication – many hospitals had their own pharmacies and an apothecary to mix the medicines.

However, the dissolution of the monasteries* in England in 1536 dramatically changed the availability of hospital care in England.

Key term

The dissolution of the monasteries*

Henry VIII split from the Catholic Church in 1533 and created the Church of England. In 1536, he disbanded certain religious institutions, such as monasteries and convents, and confiscated their land.

Since the vast majority of hospitals were connected to the Church, very few were able to stay open after the dissolution of the monasteries. As hospitals were attached to abbeys, monasteries and convents, it was the nuns and monks who administered the medical care. With the convents and monasteries gone, the hospitals also went. Saint Bartholomew's hospital in London, which was founded in 1123, only survived because Henry VIII re-founded it himself in 1546.

Some smaller hospitals opened to fill the gap left by the dissolution of the monasteries, funded by charities, but there was a big change in the amount of medical treatment provided by hospitals.

Many hospitals reopened without their religious sponsors. However, it took a long time for the amount of hospitals to return to what it had been before the dissolution of the monasteries.

Pest houses

One change in hospital care in this period was the appearance of hospitals that specialised in one particular disease. Versions of these existed in the Middle Ages, when there were lazar houses for people suffering from leprosy. There was a growing understanding that disease could be transmitted from person to person (even though people didn't understand how or why this happened). This meant that new types of hospital began to appear that catered only for people suffering from plague or pox. These were known as **pest houses**, **plague houses** or **poxhouses**.

These new types of hospital provided a much-needed service. Traditional hospitals would not admit patients who were contagious, but people suffering from serious, contagious diseases had to go somewhere or risk infecting their families.

Community care

In spite of changes to hospitals, most sick people continued to be cared for at home. Local communities were very close-knit, which meant that there were plenty of people around to give advice and even mix remedies.

Women continued to play an important role in the care of the sick. This included rich and well-born ladies like Lady Grace Mildmay (1552–1620), who kept detailed notes of the healing and treatment she carried out. It also included poor women working in big cities to support their families. We don't know a great deal about these women, but we know that a lot of them were prosecuted by the London College of Physicians for practising medicine without a licence. They usually mixed and sold simple herbal remedies to purge the body or cure a particular ailment. Records suggest that they were very popular, probably because they were cheaper than going to a licensed physician or apothecary.

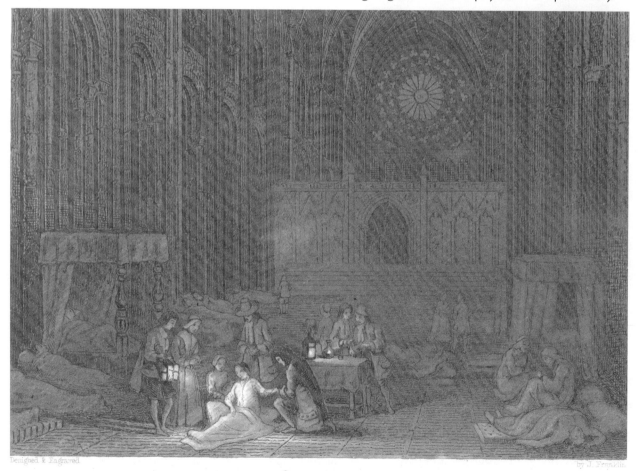

Designed & Engraved

by J. Franklin

Saint Paul's converted into a Pest House.

Figure 2.4 This 19th-century English engraving of St Paul's Cathedral shows it being used as a pest house during the Great Plague of London. St Paul's became a pest house during many outbreaks of disease in the city of London.

Interpretation 1

In this extract from an article in the *Bulletin of the History of Medicine* (2008), Deborah E. Harkness describes the attitudes of male medical professionals towards female healers in the 16th century. She suggests that we can see they were popular because male physicians at the time were very critical of them.

The view of women's medical work in London that emerges from urban records... stands in stark contrast to the view conveyed... at the same time by male medical practitioners – namely, the records of proceedings at the College of Physicians, the reports of the Barber-Surgeons' Company, and various printed works. In 1566, for example, physician John Securis surveyed the medical practitioners available to eager Elizabethan consumers – and he did not like what he saw... "presumptuous" women offended his sense of proper medical order. Securis was not alone in his opinion that women and medical work were a problematic combination. A year earlier, John Hall, an eminent Maidstone surgeon who moved to London in the 1560s, described in print how the "true minister" of surgery and the hard-working physician had to compete in the streets with the "smiths, cutlers, carters, cobblers, coopers, curriers of leather, and a great rabble of women" for the attention of potential patients.

Summary

- Methods of treatment mainly stayed the same between 1500 and 1700. Bleeding, purging and other humoural treatments were still popular. Herbal remedies were very common.
- New herbal remedies appeared. Exploration to places previously unknown, like the New World, meant that new plants were available.
- There was a new focus on chemical cures. This was known as iatrochemistry. This reflected a new interest in minerals and chemicals in society.
- People still believed in the importance of cleanliness and tried to avoid miasmata.
- Apothecaries and surgeons continued to treat the sick and received more formal training.
- By 1700, physicians studied anatomy and botany alongside their traditional medical courses.
- Vesalius, an anatomy professor, published an anatomy textbook called *On the Fabric of the Human Body*. It corrected many of Galen's mistakes and encouraged physicians to carry out their own dissections.
- Hospitals had more focus on medical treatment by the end of this period, but there were fewer of them in England because of the dissolution of the monasteries. However, the vast majority of sick people continued to be treated at home by women.

Checkpoint

Strengthen

S1 Describe the changes in the way that physicians were trained between c1250–c1500 and c1500–c1700.

S2 List five of the mistakes Vesalius found in the works of Galen.

S3 Describe the different places that sick people could seek medical treatment between 1500 and 1700.

Challenge

C1 Attitudes in society were a big factor in both driving and limiting the amount of change in treatment during this period. Select information to show three ways that people's beliefs and suspicions encouraged medical development, and three ways that they held them back.

C2 Explain the differences between hospital and community care in the period c1250–c1500 and in the period c1500–c1700.

How confident do you feel about your answers to these questions? Share your answers with a partner and see if you can improve them together.

2.3 William Harvey

Learning outcomes

- Understand the importance William Harvey's research had on anatomical knowledge.

William Harvey was born in 1578. He studied medicine at Cambridge, and then at the famous medical school in Padua. In 1615, he became a lecturer of anatomy at the College of Physicians, and by 1618 he was one of the royal doctors for James I.

Harvey had a keen interest in dissection and observing the human body, in order to improve his knowledge of human anatomy. Carrying out public dissections was part of his job. He taught his students that it was important to observe the body and believe what they saw, rather than believing what had been written in classical texts. This idea was also followed by Thomas Sydenham, who would work on this theory later that century.

Harvey's research

Harvey was particularly interested in blood. During his studies at Padua, his professors had taught him Vesalius's theory that the veins of the body contained valves, which was proof that the blood in those veins flowed towards the heart. Using dissected bodies, Harvey saw the evidence to prove this theory. When he tried to pump liquids through the veins the other way, it did not work. This proved that the blood only flowed towards the heart, contradicting what Galen had taught about the blood (see page 17).

(see page 17)

Source A

This source shows an illustration from Harvey's book, *An Anatomical Account of the Motion of the Heart and Blood in Animals*. In it, he is showing an experiment that proved blood flowed only in one direction.

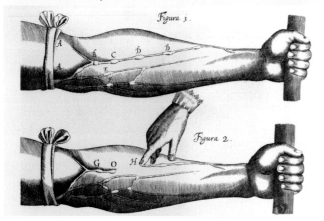

Harvey looked in more detail at the old Galenic theory. It stated that blood was made in the liver as a product of what a person ate, then flowed through the body to provide energy and was burned up. Harvey worked out that if Galen's theory was correct, the liver would have to make 1,800 litres of blood a day for a person to survive!

Harvey was influenced by new inventions that had appeared during the Renaissance. Fire engines now used mechanical pumps to provide water to put out fires: perhaps the human body worked in the same way.

Discovering the circulation of the blood

Harvey's research involved dissecting human corpses and cutting open cold-blooded animals, which had a much slower heartbeat, to observe the movement of their blood while they were still alive. Through his research, he famously proved that arteries and veins were linked together into one system. This was done by tying a tight cord around somebody's arm and cutting off the blood flow in the artery leading into the arm. Because the artery in the arm is deeper than the veins, loosening the cord a little bit allowed blood to flow into the arm but stopped it from flowing out and the veins swelled with blood. Harvey's theory was that blood must pass from arteries to veins through tiny passages that were invisible to the naked eye. Today we know about these blood vessels – they are called capillaries.

Galen had suggested that blood flowed from one side of the heart to the other through invisible pores in the walls of the ventricles. He also said that veins carried both blood and pneuma*, which was picked up in the lungs, while arteries carried just blood. Harvey's theory criticised both of these ideas. He showed that the veins carried only blood. He proved that the heart acted as a pump just as the new mechanical fire pumps did.

Key word

Pneuma*

Means 'breath of life'. Galen thought it was both the air that you breathe and your life force, or soul.

Factors enabling Harvey's discoveries

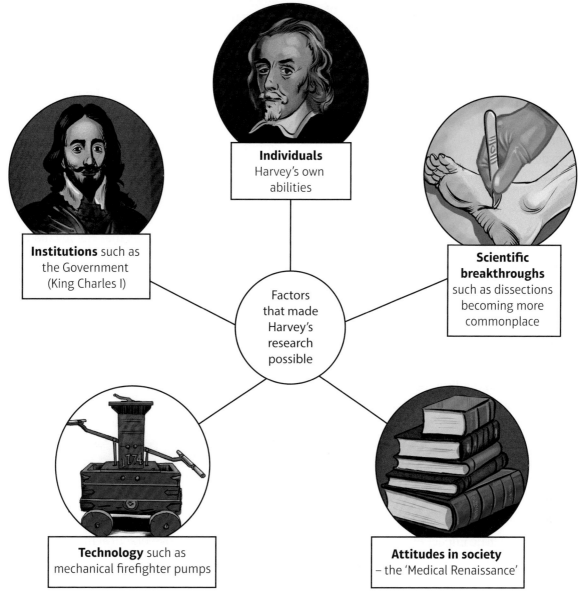

Figure 2.5 Five factors enabling Harvey's discoveries.

Individuals and institutions

Individuals such as Vesalius had previously proved parts of the work of Galen wrong, which made it easier for other scientists and physicians to do the same.

Harvey was employed by Charles I as his personal physician. This gave him credibility, in the same way the royal charter gave credibility to the Royal Society (see page 46). More people heard of Harvey's theory about the circulation of blood.

The decline of the power of the Church also enabled Harvey to be critical of Galen's teachings.

Science and technology

Newly popular technologies, like the pump used when fighting fires, inspired Harvey to look again at how the heart worked.

Attitudes in society

There was more interest in science and in solving some of the puzzles of the human body. People had begun to search for rational explanations for things.

The impact of Harvey

Harvey's arguments relied on careful observations of human and animal anatomy. Many people consider his book, *An Anatomical Account of the Motion of the Heart and Blood in Animals,* to be the beginning of modern physiology. However, Harvey did not consider himself to be a 'modern' scientist. He didn't believe many of Galen's theories, but he did follow the teachings of another classical thinker: Aristotle. Like Aristotle, he believed that the body was designed by a higher power, and thought that the soul was responsible for how the body worked.

The most immediate impact that Harvey's theory had was to encourage other scientists to experiment on actual bodies. For example, Harvey had proved that the liver did not digest food to create blood. If the liver didn't make blood, what did it do? Harvey had proved that blood circulated, instead of being absorbed to provide nourishment for the body – how, then, was the body nourished?

However, understanding the circulation of the blood had little practical use in medical treatment. This meant that the impact of Harvey's discoveries on treatment during the 17th century was quite limited. He may have paved the way for a modern understanding of anatomy and how the human body functions, but a lot of doctors at the time ignored him. Some even openly criticised him. Nobody liked to be told that they had been doing their job incorrectly. They also reasoned that nobody recovered from disease by simply knowing that the blood flowed to the heart. To many, it had no practical application. English medical textbooks continued to give Galen's account until 1651; Harvey's ideas only began to appear in universities from 1673.

Activities

1. Draw an outline of a person. Label it with the different discoveries that Harvey made about the human body and blood.

2. Like Vesalius, Harvey is a key individual who had an impact on medicine. Create a fact file about him to use in revision. You should include: details of his background, his experiments and his impact on medicine.

3. Write a short paragraph to explain why Harvey's work did not have much impact when it was first published.

Summary

- William Harvey discovered that blood circulated around the body, instead of being made in the liver and absorbed into the body, as previously theorised by Galen.
- Harvey also proved that the heart acted as a pump, propelling blood around the body.
- Harvey's work had little impact at first, because it couldn't be used to improve practical medical treatments.
- Harvey inspired other scientists to carry out further experiments, building on his discoveries about blood and circulation.

Checkpoint

Strengthen

S1 Name three discoveries that Harvey made.

S2 Describe the methods Harvey used to investigate his theories.

S3 What was Harvey's biggest impact in the short term?

Challenge

C1 Think back to the factors that affect change and continuity in medicine. How many of them can you link to the history of Harvey?

C2 Who had the biggest impact on ideas about the human body – Vesalius or Harvey? Select information from this chapter to support your argument.

To help structure your answer to C2, you might find it useful to create a 'For' and 'Against' list for both individuals.

In 1665, a serious outbreak of the plague swept across the whole of England. Lasting from June until November, the rate of infection of the Great Plague peaked in September, when 7,000 deaths from the disease were recorded in one week. Across the whole outbreak, 100,000 Londoners died – one in five people. It was the last serious outbreak of the disease in England, but people were as helpless to resist it as they had been over 300 years earlier. As with previous epidemics, the disease was spread by fleas carried on rats.

Ideas about the causes of the Great Plague

Although fewer people believed in the Theory of the Four Humours by 1665, it had not been replaced with any proven alternative. Still, nobody knew for certain what caused disease in general. Therefore, most people blamed the same things for the Great Plague in 1665 as they had during the Black Death in 1348.

Astrology

There had been an unusual alignment between Saturn and Jupiter in October 1664, and between Mars and Saturn on 12 November. These were seen as unlucky combinations that suggested there was trouble ahead. Worse still, a comet had been spotted, too.

Punishment from God

Many people believed the Great Plague was a result of mankind's wickedness and that God had sent it to clean up his kingdom.

Miasma

In contrast to the Black Death outbreak in 1348, by far the most popular theory about the spread of the Great Plague in 1665 was that it was caused by a miasma.

People believed this miasma had been created by the stinking rubbish and dunghills that were a feature of 17th-century city life. The vapour was present in the soil, where it would stay as long as the weather stayed cold. When the weather turned warmer, however, the vapour would pour out of the earth as a plague-carrying miasma. This fitted the pattern of the infection: plague outbreaks generally appeared when the weather began to turn warmer.

Other people

By 1665, many people believed the correct idea that disease could be spread from person to person, although, as there was no proof that this was the case it was not the most popular theory. However, plague victims were still quarantined. Even people who believed a miasma caused the disease believed that, once people had caught it, they could pass it on to others.

Approaches to treatment of the Great Plague

We don't know a great deal about treatments that were given to plague victims in 1665. This is partly because so many of them were shut up with family members in quarantine, so there are not many records of the methods they attempted to keep people alive.

We do know that some of the new ideas about treatment of diseases had an impact on plague treatments in 1665. As was the fashion at the time, physicians advised that patients be wrapped in thick woollen cloths and laid by a fire so that they could sweat the disease out. Transference was also a popular idea – methods such as strapping a live chicken to a bubo, or lancing it with a feather plucked from a live chicken, were meant to draw out the poison and help the patient to recover.

Recipes for herbal remedies continued to be extremely popular. These took the form of medicines, poultices or rubs.

Quack doctors* took advantage of the general panic. They mixed remedies and advertised them as fabulous cures, hoping to make some easy money.

Key term

Quack doctor*

Somebody who did not have any medical qualifications, but who sold their services as a doctor or apothecary.

Source A

This recipe from Culpeper's *Complete Herbal* is for a 17th-century version of medieval theriaca. It was known as London treacle and was a popular treatment for, and preventative against, the plague.

Take ... the seeds of citrons, sorrel, peony, basil, of each one ounce; scoridum, coraliana, of each six drams; the roots of angelica, tormentil, peony, the leaves of dittany, bay-berries, juniper berries, of each half an ounce; the flowers of rosemary, marigolds, clove, gilliflowers, the tops of St John's wort, nutmegs, saffron, of each three drams; the roots of gentian, zedoary, ginger, mace, myrrh, the leaves of scabious, devil's-bit, carduus, of each two drams; cloves, opium, of each a dram; Malaga wine as much is sufficient ... mix them according to art.

People still did not understand the cause of the Great Plague and therefore could not treat it effectively. The best advice was the same as it had always been: make sure you don't catch it in the first place.

Approaches to preventing the Great Plague

Advice from physicians

The College of Physicians recommended a variety of preventative measures that could be taken to avoid catching the Great Plague.

- Prayer and repentance
- Quarantine anybody who had the plague.
- Carrying a pomander was a way to drive away miasma. A pomander was a ball containing perfumed substances.
- Various diets were suggested, from eating almost nothing (fasting) to eating a diet heavy with garlic and sage fried in butter.
- Plague doctors wore special costumes to avoid catching the plague from their patients. They had hooked, birdlike masks, with sweet-smelling herbs to ward off the miasma. Birds were meant to attract disease, so it was thought that the disease might be attracted to the bird shape and leave the patient. More practically, the physician's cloak would be treated with wax to make sure that none of the pus or blood from the patient soaked into it.

Advice from other healers

Most people turned to local healers for help in warding off the plague. Recipes for plague water, a 'treatment' for the plague, were popular among apothecaries. Some relied on native herbs that would have been used in England for centuries, such as mint and rosemary, while others contained new, exotic ingredients such as nutmeg and sugar. Smoking tobacco was encouraged to ward off the miasma.

Some people thought that, because buboes were symptoms of both syphilis and the Great Plague, catching syphilis would prevent a person from catching the Great Plague. They went out of their way to become infected with syphilis – though this, of course, did not prevent them catching the Great Plague.

Government action

Local governments also tried to prevent the plague from spreading. Unlike the first large outbreak of the plague, this time they did more, and so did the king. Charles II decreed that people should fast regularly and made a list of actions to try to stop the spread of the plague. These were carried out by local government officials of each city, including the mayor. Public meetings, fairs and even large funerals were banned. Theatres were closed. Streets and alleyways were swept and cleaned. Fires were set to burn on street corners, often in barrels of tar or strewn with sweet-smelling herbs, to drive away the evil miasma. Cats, dogs and pigeons were killed if they were seen on the street. Around 40,000 dogs and 200,000 cats were slaughtered because people thought they were helping to spread the disease.

The mayor also appointed searchers and wardens to monitor the spread of the disease. Searchers would go from house to house, checking to see if there were any plague victims in each one. If a household was infected, the inhabitants were either taken to the pest house or quarantined inside the house for 40 days. The house was painted with a red cross together with the words, 'Lord have mercy on us'. The parish officials were in charge of bringing them food and other necessities. Every day, carts would travel through the city to collect the bodies of the dead.

Many people believed the best way to avoid the Great Plague, was the same as it had been in 1348: run away. People in 1665 still did not know what caused the plague, but they realised that this ignorance could kill them. Since there was no known cure for the disease, people focused on prevention, since methods of prevention had been successful in the past. Rather than attempt wild treatments, they put their energy into stopping the disease from spreading, or into escaping it completely.

Exam-style question, Section B

Explain **one** way in which ideas about preventing the plague were different in the 14th and 17th centuries.

4 marks

Exam tip

The Black Death of 1348 and the Great Plague of 1665 are both case studies for this unit. That means that the examiner will want to see that you recognise the similarities and differences between these two specific outbreaks.

Source B

In this engraving from 1665, you can see how people reacted to the Great Plague: by fleeing London and burying the dead.

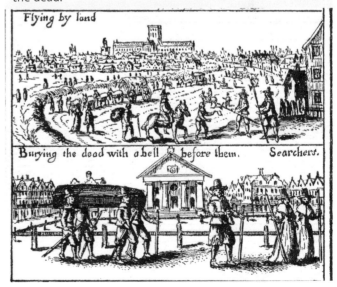

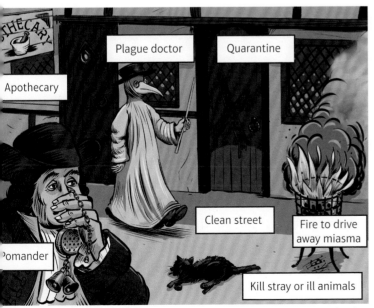

Figure 2.6 A 17th-century street showing different methods used to prevent the Great Plague.

THINKING HISTORICALLY ▸ Change and continuity (2b)

Events or historical change?

Change is an alteration in a situation. Events are when something happens.

Sometimes a situation can be very different before and after an event – this event **marks a change**.

However, sometimes a situation is the same before and after an event, and sometimes a situation changes without a specific event taking place at all.

Study the following events and their changes:

The English Reformation reduced the power of the Church.	Vesalius published *On the Fabric of the Human Body*.	The Royal Society was founded in 1660.	The ideas of Galen slowly became discredited.
Careful observation of patients became more important when diagnosing disease.	Most people now recognised that God did not send disease.	Thomas Sydenham published *Observationes Medicae*	Improved communications enabled scientists to study each other's research.

1 Sort the above into 'events' and 'changes'.

2 Match each event to the change that it marks.

3 In your own words, describe what the difference is between an event and a change.

4 Can you think of any historical change that has happened without there being a particular event associated with it?

Summary

- Causes of the Great Plague were thought to be supernatural – either to do with the planets or as a punishment from God – or caused by a miasma.
- Most people now recognised that the plague was spread from person to person.
- Prevention methods often involved creating a strong smell to ward off the miasma.
- The local government in London took a lot more action than in previous outbreaks.

Checkpoint

Strengthen

S1 Create a mnemonic to help you remember what people thought caused the Great Plague – Astrology, God, Miasma and Other People.

S2 What did quack doctors do during the Great Plague?

Challenge

C1 How did a change in attitudes in society and the role of the Church lead to changes in the way the plague was tackled between 1348 and 1665? Hint: in 1665 there was more focus on prevention than there had been before.

C2 Can you identify three changes and three continuities between the case studies of the Black Death and the Great Plague?

If you are not sure, go back to the text in this section to find the details you need.

Recap: The Medical Renaissance in England, c1500–c1700

Activity **?**

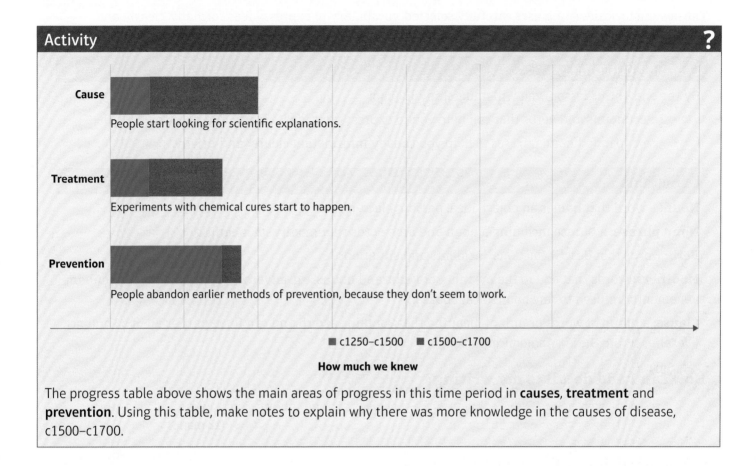

Cause

People start looking for scientific explanations.

Treatment

Experiments with chemical cures start to happen.

Prevention

People abandon earlier methods of prevention, because they don't seem to work.

■ c1250–c1500 ■ c1500–c1700

How much we knew

The progress table above shows the main areas of progress in this time period in **causes**, **treatment** and **prevention**. Using this table, make notes to explain why there was more knowledge in the causes of disease, c1500–c1700.

Recall quiz

1 Name three doctors who came up with new theories about the causes of illness in this period.

2 Why was Thomas Sydenham important to medical progress in the 17th century?

3 What was invented in around 1440 that helped the spread of scientific knowledge?

4 What was the name of the Royal Society's science journal?

5 What is iatrochemistry?

6 Why did people take fewer baths in the 1500s?

7 Roughly how many mistakes did Vesalius find in the works of Galen?

8 Where were plague victims sent for treatment?

9 Who proved that blood circulated within the body?

10 List two ways in which people attempted to prevent the spread of the Great Plague.

Exam-style question, Section B ○

Explain why there was continuity in the way disease was treated in the period c1500–c1700.

You may use the following information in your answer:

• the Great Plague

• attitudes in society.

You **must** also use information of your own. **12 marks**

Exam tip ○

What you leave out of an exam answer is as much a message to the examiner as what you include. Make sure all your information supports your answer to the question. Don't make the mistake of writing down everything you can think of: this is a clear sign of somebody who doesn't know the significance of the facts and is trying to hide it.

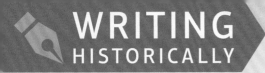
Writing historically: selecting vocabulary

The best historical writing uses carefully selected vocabulary to express ideas formally, clearly and precisely.

Learning outcomes

By the end of this lesson, you will understand how to:

- select nouns and verbs that can help you to express your ideas clearly and precisely
- use expanded noun phrases to help you convey information clearly and briefly.

Definitions

Noun: a word that names an object, idea, person, place, etc.

Noun phrase: a phrase including a noun and any words that modify its meaning.

Verb: words that describe actions, incidents and situations

Modifiers: words that add to the meaning of verbs and nouns, e.g. adverbs, adjectives, etc. ('Sydenham vehemently refused to rely on medical books').

Clause: a group of words or unit of meaning that contains a verb and can form part or all of a sentence ('Vesalius wrote the *Six Anatomical Tables*').

How can I add detail to my writing?

> Explain why there were changes in the way ideas about the cause of disease and illness were communicated in the period c1500–c1700. **(12 marks)**

Look at the first sentence of one response to the above exam-style question. The key nouns, verbs and modifiers in the sentence have been highlighted:

> The microscope showed small 'animalcules', which helped to question the thoughts of others.

1. How could you improve this sentence? Would you add more detail? Or would you express the same information more formally and precisely? Or would you do both?

2. Rewrite the sentence using more precise nouns, verbs and modifiers. You could use the thesaurus extracts below to help you.

showed	small	helped	question	thoughts	others
revealed	tiny	assisted	disprove	theories	contemporaries
unmasked	microscopic	allowed	challenge	ideas	conservatives
discovered	miniscule	enabled	test	wisdom	rivals
demonstrated	miniature	facilitated	contest	explanations	other doctors

Now look at the next two sentences from the same response.

> Better pictures meant that more and more things could be found. These findings could be shared in books by other people.

a. Identify all the nouns, verbs and modifiers.

b. For each noun, verb or modifier, note down two or three alternative choices.

c. Rewrite the sentences above, choosing more formal, precise nouns, verbs and modifiers.

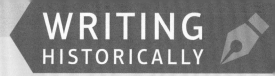

How can I make the information in my writing clear and concise?

One way in which you can make your writing more concise is by using **expanded noun phrases**.

Compare these two versions of the same sentence from a response to the exam-style question on the previous page.

> The microscope revealed small 'animalcules' and challenged previous theories.

> The microscope's revelations were a challenge to previous theories.

The second sentence expresses the same ideas and information much more clearly and concisely.

3. Look at another sentence from this response to the exam-style question on the previous page:

> The Royal Society held meetings of fellow scientists and this encouraged greater sharing.

a. Experiment with different ways of rewriting the sentence by condensing the highlighted clause to form an expanded noun phrase.

b. Compare your rewritten sentences with the original version. Which version do you prefer? Write a sentence or two explaining your decision.

Did you notice?

4. In the examples above, the shorter noun phrase has been created by turning a verb into a noun. Copy and complete the table below, turning the verbs into nouns. The first two have been done to help you.

Verbs	Nouns
to reveal	revelation
to challenge	challenge
to introduce	
to create	
to submit	
to accept	

Improving an answer

5. Now look at the next section of this response:

> The society published its book in 1665. It contained ideas written by other people. This helped to share what they did and did lots for spreading ideas. They also turned other books into English so everyone could read them. They put their work together in a library. This meant people could read each other's work and was therefore good for starting new ideas.

a. Improve the sentences by replacing nouns, verbs and modifiers with more formal and precise vocabulary.

b. Now experiment with different ways of rewriting the sentences, using expanded noun phrases to make them more concise. Start by looking at each verb and seeing whether you can convert it to a noun.

c. Look at all the different versions you have written of this response. Which version is clearest and most concise? Write a sentence or two explaining your decision.

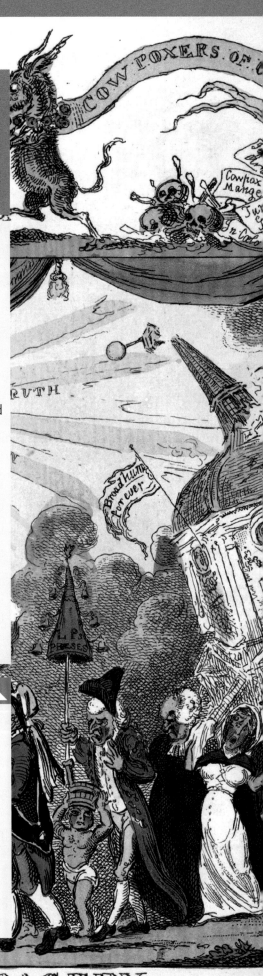

03 | c1700–c1900: Medicine in 18th- and 19th-century Britain

From the start of the 18th century, rapid changes began to occur in medicine. Between 1500 and 1700, many new medical theories had been published: however, it was not until later that those theories were put into practice.

At the start of the period c1700–c1900, the Theory of the Four Humours was no longer widely believed, but it had not yet been replaced by anything else. Bleeding and purging were still common treatments. Apothecaries still sold herbal remedies and most treatment was still carried out by women in the home. Luckily, epidemic diseases such as the plague seemed to have disappeared, but smallpox and other diseases were common.

By 1900, the medical landscape had been completely transformed. Germs had been discovered, and there was ongoing work to create vaccines and develop treatments for the disease caused by them.

Edward Jenner had developed the first vaccination for smallpox – and a British government more willing to get involved in day-to-day life had made this vaccination compulsory in 1852.

Hospitals had been developed into clean, modern institutions, thanks to the work of Florence Nightingale. Developments in **anaesthetics** and **antiseptics** meant that surgery was now much less dangerous, and therefore much more common.

This was an incredibly exciting period in the history of medicine: a time when all the ideas and theories of the past came together to change the way patients were diagnosed and treated.

Learning outcomes

By the end of Chapter 3, you will:

- understand what ideas people in Britain c1700–c1900 had about the causes of disease and illness, and how these had changed from previous periods
- recognise the impact of the work of Pasteur and Koch on people's understanding of the causes of disease and illness
- understand what methods people used to treat disease in 18th- and 19th-century Britain
- understand the ways in which people attempted to prevent disease including vaccinations and the work of Edward Jenner, and government action and the work of John Snow.

THE COW POX TRAGEDY

3.1 Ideas about the cause of disease and illness

Learning outcomes

- Understand how ideas about the cause of disease changed and stayed the same, 1700–1900.

The 18th century was a very exciting time in the world of science. In 1700, the influence of the Church was not as great as it once was. Many people no longer believed that God was responsible for all worldly events. Instead, they focused on developing scientific explanations. Intellectual movements such as the Enlightenment* made it fashionable to seek answers to questions about the world – including disease and illness.

Key term

The Enlightenment*

A movement in Europe during the 18th century that promoted the idea that people could think for themselves and that traditional authorities, like the nobility and the Church, should not be able to control everyday life.

This fashion for rational explanations touched every part of life – politics, philosophy, history, economics and, of course, science. In fact, the 'Age of Enlightenment' was happening at the same time as the Scientific Revolution, during which developments across all branches of science completely changed the way people lived and the ways they understood the world around them.

Some historians suggest that there were two halves to the Scientific Revolution.

- In the first half, starting with the Renaissance in the 16th century, old theories were discredited.
- In the second half, new ideas began to replace the old. This half of the Scientific Revolution began in c1700.

Society itself was also changing. Cities began to grow as people moved there in search of jobs. The new cities were not well planned and quickly became dirty and disease-ridden. Diseases like tuberculosis, typhus and smallpox were a big threat to this new working population. Therefore, understanding the causes of disease and illness became even more important.

Continuity and change

There were not a lot of new ideas about the causes of disease in the 18th century. Ideas such as the Theory of the Four Humours had been discarded. People still believed in miasma, although this theory was also becoming less popular.

Scientists in the early 18th century developed the theory of **spontaneous generation** as an alternative to theories like the Four Humours. Improvements in the quality of the glass lenses used in microscopes meant that scientists could see microbes* present on decaying matter*. Most people believed that these microbes were the **product** of decay, rather than the **cause** of it.

Key terms

Microbes*

A microbe is any living organism that is too small to see without a microscope. Microbes include bacteria.

Decaying matter*

Material, such as vegetables or animals, that has died and is rotting.

In the 18th century, this was just a theory, and scientists were unable to prove that spontaneous generation was correct. It took until the 19th century for scientists to make a solid link between these microbes and disease.

Medical breakthrough: Germ Theory

Louis Pasteur and the development of Germ Theory

In 1860, the French Academy of Science challenged scientists to come up with evidence to either prove or disprove the theory of spontaneous generation.

By the middle of the 19th century, microscopes had improved even more – it was now possible to magnify substances to a much higher level and keep the image clear enough to see. Because of this, Louis Pasteur, a French scientist, was able to observe unwanted microbes in wine and vinegar, which turned both liquids 'bad'.

Pasteur published the results of his experiments in 1861. He called his discovery **Germ Theory**.

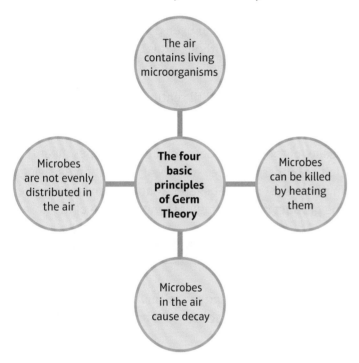

Figure 3.1 The four basic principles of Germ Theory.

Extend your knowledge

Germs

Pasteur called the microorganisms he observed 'germs' because he observed the microorganisms growing, or germinating.

Pasteur proved that the idea of spontaneous generation was wrong because decay did not happen to sterilised matter that was left undisturbed. Instead, something in the air was causing the decay.

Pasteur also theorised that, as germs were causing decay, they might also be causing disease in the human body. He observed one particular type of microorganism killing off France's silkworm population, which seemed to prove this theory. However, he did not publish this **germ theory of infection** until 1878.

Pasteur's influence in Britain

To begin with, Pasteur's work had almost no impact on British ideas about the causes of illness and disease. He was not a doctor, and his work focused on decay and spoiled food, not disease.

In Britain, the theory of spontaneous generation continued to be important until the 1870s. It was promoted by Dr Henry Bastian, who was one of the most powerful doctors in the country. Because he was so well-respected, few people disagreed with him.

However, some scientists did start to look for a link between the microbes and disease. One of these was Joseph Lister, who read Pasteur's germ theory and linked it to the infection problems his surgical patients had experienced (see page 82).

Another scientist who promoted the link between microbes and disease was John Tyndall. He had discovered that there were small organic* particles in the air. In January 1870, he gave a lecture, linking his discovery with Pasteur's germ theory and Lister's work on wound infection. Tyndall theorised that dust particles carried the germs that caused disease.

Key term

Organic*

Something that is living or that has once been alive.

However, Tyndall was not a doctor: he was a physicist. The medical world trusted Bastian's beliefs rather than Tyndall's theory.

Lister's ideas were also doubted, as he could not prove his theory. Although microscopes meant that microbes were visible, there were lots of them present in the blood or in a wound. Doctors could not yet identify what they were and what role they played. The gut is a good example of why they had problems: when examined under the microscope, scientists saw hundreds of microbes, even in healthy people. It seemed impossible to people that these microbes caused disease, too (see Source A).

Source A

In this extract from an article published in the *British Medical Journal* in 1875, Dr Henry Bastian explains why he does not believe microbes (bacteria) cause disease.

```
Bacteria... habitually exist in so many
parts of the body in every human being...
as to make it almost inconceivable that
these organisms can be causes of disease.
In support of this statement I have only to
say, that even in a healthy person they may
be found in myriads... the whole alimentary
tract from mouth to anus; they exist
throughout the air-passages, and may be found
in mucus coming from the nasal cavities...
They exist... within the skin, not only in
the face, but in other parts of the body.
Fresh legions of them are being introduced...
with almost every meal that is taken.
```

Therefore, Pasteur's theory had limited impact in Britain, because **attitudes among doctors** meant people refused to recognise the link between germs and disease – even though the link was correct.

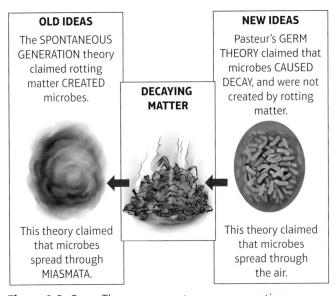

OLD IDEAS	DECAYING MATTER	NEW IDEAS
The SPONTANEOUS GENERATION theory claimed rotting matter CREATED microbes.		Pasteur's GERM THEORY claimed that microbes CAUSED DECAY, and were not created by rotting matter.
This theory claimed that microbes spread through MIASMATA.		This theory claimed that microbes spread through the air.

Figure 3.2 Germ Theory vs. spontaneous generation.

Robert Koch's work on microbes

Pasteur had been the first scientist to identify microbes and their role in decay. However, it was the German scientist Robert Koch who successfully identified that different germs cause many common diseases.

Koch discovered the bacteria that caused tuberculosis, in 1882. He then published his ideas on the methods that could be used to identify disease-causing microbes.

1   The microbe is present in every case of the disease.

2   Once taken from the body, the microbe can be reproduced into a pure culture*.

3   The disease can be reproduced in test animals using that culture.

4   The microbe can be taken out of the test animals and used to start a fresh culture.

Key term

Culture*
Bacteria grown under controlled conditions.

Koch continued to look for the microbes causing different diseases. In 1883, he discovered cholera, and in 1884 he proved that it was spread in water supplies when he found it in the drinking water in India, where a cholera epidemic had broken out. This also provided proof for John Snow's theory (see page 92).

Koch made it easier for future scientists to study bacteria by developing a new method of growing them, using agar jelly in a petri dish. This made it easier to study the bacteria under a microscope. Later, Koch also developed a method for staining them with industrial dyes, to make them easier to see.

Koch's research inspired other scientists. Over the next two decades, they went on to discover the microbes responsible for other diseases, such as diphtheria, pneumonia, meningitis, the plague, tetanus and various other infections. Koch received the Nobel Prize for Medicine in 1905. He is considered to be the father of bacteriology* and his methods are still used when seeking out the microbes responsible for disease today.

Key term

Bacteriology*
The study of bacteria.

Source B

In this cartoon from 1880, Robert Koch is likened to St George. The saddle is labelled 'Investigation' and he is using a microscope as a weapon to slay tuberculosis, the snake.

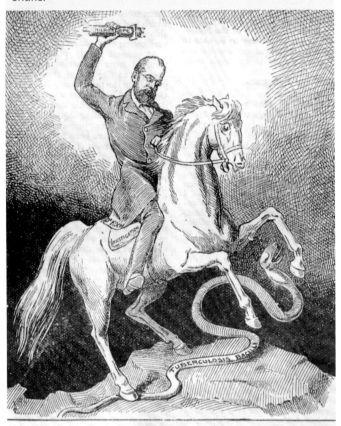

KOCH AS THE NEW ST. GEORGE.

Koch's influence in Britain

The identification of microbes that caused particular diseases was an enormous breakthrough in the diagnosis of disease. Whereas before, doctors had studied and treated symptoms, now they studied the disease itself. The medical profession had begun to recognise that the microbe created the symptoms of the disease, and it was the microbe that needed to be removed.

For example, in 1883, the microbe that caused diphtheria was found. Diphtheria was a horrible disease that mostly affected children. It caused a painful cough and a fever. A leathery skin would grow over the tonsils and the back of the throat, which meant that the sufferer could not breathe. By studying the microbe, scientists were able to observe that it produced a poison. The poison, when breathed, stayed in the throat and caused the painful symptoms. Since the microbe had been identified,

scientists were able to seek ways of attacking it directly, rather than just treating the symptoms.

Extend your knowledge

Sceptics of the germ theory of disease

Many doctors remained sceptical about the link between germs and disease. One Munich chemist, Max von Pettenkofer, asked Koch for a sample of the cholera microbes, which he then drank. Amazingly, he did not develop cholera – it is likely that the germs were killed off by his stomach acid. Stunts like this did nothing to help convince people that cholera was spread through dirty water.

Summary: the impact of Germ Theory in Britain

Progress in treatment and prevention using Germ Theory was slow. Once Pasteur, Koch and other scientists had found the specific disease-causing microbes, cures and vaccines could be tested. Only after this did Germ Theory begin to have a direct impact on medical treatment.

Even the British government rejected the Germ Theory of disease at first. When Koch travelled to Calcutta in 1884 to study an outbreak of cholera, he proved that it was caused by microbes in the supply of drinking water. However, this was ignored by the British government. Instead, they kept to the idea that the disease was present in the soil, and the miasma was brought out by the weather. This seemed to make sense, since there was more cholera around during the rainy season.

Despite these setbacks, in the 20th century Germ Theory and the new study of bacteriology had an enormous impact on our understanding of the causes of disease and illness. It is now recognised that many diseases are caused by a microorganism – bacteria, virus or fungus. When diagnosing disease, doctors now look for symptoms and try to match them to a disease caused by a specific microbe.

By the end of the 19th century, the mystery around what caused illness and disease had been solved. It took a little more time for this to be accepted by the medical profession, but the evidence had been found. Now it was time to start looking for new treatments based on this new science.

Interpretation 1

In *Disease, Class and Social Change* (2012), Marc Arnold explains that Germ Theory only had a limited impact in Britain during the 19th century.

Many historians have attributed the growing concern with public health from the 1880s as being solely due to the advent of bacteriology, and particularly to Robert Koch's discovery of the tuberculosis bacteria in 1882. However, the impact of germ theory in England during the 19th and early 20th centuries has probably been overstated. In 1897 the physician James Lindsay, reviewing the impact of Koch's discovery in Britain, noted that most of the respondents to an investigation by the British Medical Association did not view tuberculosis as an infectious disease.

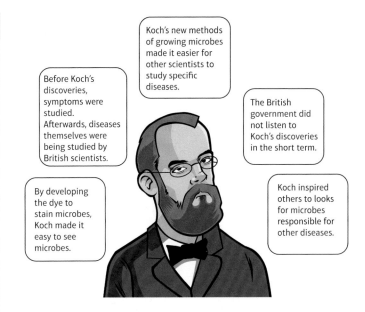

Figure 3.3 Koch's influence in Britain.

THINKING HISTORICALLY   Change and continuity (3a)

Significant change

Things change all the time. Every second something in the world is changing. If historians weighted every change as equal, they would never be able to write anything about the past that was useful. The decisions that historians make about what is historically significant and what is not is a very important part of their work.

The development of the Germ Theory of Disease

In 1861, Pasteur identified that microbes were causing decay in wine.	Dr Bastien, a very well-respected doctor, promoted the theory of spontaneous generation until his death in 1915.	In 1854, John Snow used observation to show that cholera was water-borne.	In 1882, Koch identified the microbe that caused tuberculosis.
Koch developed a new method for growing and observing bacteria.	In 1870, physicist John Tyndall theorised that disease was spread through dust particles.	Joseph Lister read Pasteur's work and linked it with infection problems in surgery.	Leeuwenhoek observed microbes and wrote to the Royal Society about them.

Imagine you are investigating how scientists' understanding of the causes of disease developed over time.

1. With a partner, discuss what might make a change significant for this investigation. E.g. how long the change lasted, or the wider consequences of the change, could affect how significant you think a change was. Write down your top three criteria.

2. Discuss your choice of criteria as a class, writing down all the suggestions. Assess your own three criteria again and decide if you want to change any of them.

3. Using your three criteria for deciding significance, put the eight changes above into order of significance, with the most significant change at the top.

4. Compare your list with that of another pair in your class. Is the order similar?

5. Compare your list of criteria affecting significance with the other pair. Does this explain why you put the changes into different orders?

6. Write a short paragraph explaining what you think makes a change significant.

Activities ?

1 Create a timeline to show the development of Germ Theory. Include events from the work of both Pasteur and Koch.

2 Create flash cards to help you revise the new theories. Create one card each for Pasteur and Koch, showing the impact they had in Britain.

3 Did Pasteur or Koch do more to improve understanding of disease? Have a debate with a partner to help you better understand the role of each scientist.

Factors affecting the understanding of the causes of illness and disease

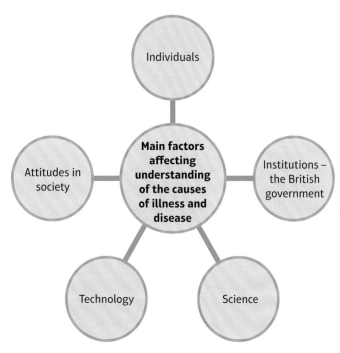

Figure 3.4 Main factors affecting understanding of the causes of illness and disease.

Individuals

The most important individuals in the development of Germ Theory were Pasteur and Koch. Without them, it might have taken a lot longer for the Germ Theory of Disease to be developed. There were also dozens of other scientists whose individual contributions helped put pieces of the puzzle into place, including John Tyndall and Joseph Lister.

Institutions: the British government

The government in Britain did not help to improve understanding of disease. For much of the 19th century, they were not interested in getting involved with everyday life. However, once more people gained the ability to vote, the government was more willing to intervene (although they were more interested in practical solutions to the problems of epidemics like cholera and typhoid). Since Germ Theory offered no practical solution to the problem of disease, they did not promote it.

Science

The second part of the Scientific Revolution focused on finding answers to the big questions of science. There was a strong desire to prove new theories and provide practical solutions to scientific problems.

Improved communication enabled scientists to share their work with each other. Scientists were able to read the work of their peers and to draw their own conclusions and theories. For example, Tyndall's 1870 theory about germs causing disease was based on the work of Pasteur and Lister. Ideas were shared across different branches of science. For example, Pasteur's work on animal diseases inspired other scientists to use his methods to diagnose human diseases.

Technology

The microscope was arguably the most important piece of technology that made the development of Germ Theory possible. Clearer images and higher magnification made it possible to spot most microorganisms, although not all – viruses, for example, are so small that they can only be seen with a very powerful microscope.

Other technological developments also helped. Koch developed a way to grow microbes. His colleague, Joseph Petri, developed the petri dish. By the end of the century, experiments with dyes had helped scientists to better observe bacteria.

Attitudes in society

Attitudes in society were both a help and a hindrance to the widespread acceptance of Germ Theory. People were more interested in finding the reasons behind disease than they had been in previous centuries.

Due to the Enlightenment, they were more interested in rational explanations for disease. Also, overcrowded cities and poor living conditions led to dangerous outbreaks of disease. Many people were horrified by the sights they saw on the street and the impact bad health had on the poor. Furthermore, an unhealthy population could not work. Religious reformers and hard-nosed businessmen agreed: something needed to be done to solve the problem of epidemics.

However, people's reluctance to change their minds slowed the spread of Germ Theory. It took a long time to show that specific microbes were always present when people were suffering from a particular disease. Until this proof was provided, from the 1880s onwards, Germ Theory did not become an accepted fact.

Exam-style question, Section B

'There was rapid change in ideas about the causes of illness and disease in the period c1700–c1900'.

How far do you agree with this statement? You may use the following information in your answer:

- Spontaneous generation
- Louis Pasteur.

You **must** also use information of your own. **16 marks**

Exam tip

Two hundred years is a long period of time. It is unlikely that rapid change would ever go on for so long. In your answer, try to pinpoint where exactly the rapid change occurred. Make sure you explain what criteria you have used to make your judgement.

Summary

- In the 18th and 19th centuries, scientists started to theorise about germs being produced by decaying matter, a theory named spontaneous generation.
- In 1861, Louis Pasteur, a French chemist, published Germ Theory. This proved that microbes in the air caused decay in substances such as wine and vinegar.
- Pasteur's work was picked up by some medical professions quite quickly, particularly in Britain where Joseph Lister began attempting to remove microbes from his operating theatre. However, many doctors resisted the ideas.
- Robert Koch, a German scientist, began to look for specific microbes that caused disease. He identified lots of these, including the microbe that caused cholera.
- By c1900, the mystery of what caused many illnesses and diseases had been solved – it was just that not everybody believed the solution yet.

Checkpoint

Strengthen

S1 Describe in detail the roles of Pasteur and Koch in developing the Germ Theory of Disease.

S2 List the four basic principles of Germ Theory.

S3 Why didn't scientists always believe Koch's ideas about microbes?

S4 How much impact did the Germ Theory have on Britain by c1900?

Challenge

C1 To begin with, Pasteur's work did not have many practical applications. Name some similar discoveries from previous periods.

C2 Which factor do you think had the biggest impact on the development of understanding about the causes of disease and illness? Explain why you think this.

If you are struggling with these questions, ask your teacher for some hints.

Learning outcomes

- Understand how approaches to prevention and treatment changed and stayed the same, c1700–c1900.

The extent of change in care and treatment

By 1900, the way that sick people were treated and cared for had changed almost completely since 1700. However, there was some continuity in treatment because it took a while for medical science to catch up to the new ideas about the causes of illness and disease. By 1900, most people accepted that germs caused disease and that treatment needed to be focused on removing the germ. Unfortunately, there was still not a great deal of understanding about how best to do this. Scientists were working incredibly hard to come up with treatments for everyday diseases such as syphilis and tuberculosis, but it was not until after 1900 that these were successfully developed. Therefore, old herbal remedies continued to be popular.

Similarly, by 1900, the old belief that prevention was the most important aspect became even more widespread. People began to realise that infection was everywhere: on dirty clothes, medical instruments and unwashed hands, and in the air and water. The old idea of avoiding disease by keeping clean and following a sanitary regime suddenly made sense, because people really did need to protect themselves against something invisible.

Perhaps the biggest change by 1900 was in the **willingness of the government and the population to take steps to prevent disease from spreading.**

Activities ?

1. Create a spider diagram to show changes and continuities in treatments by c1900.
2. Next to each label on your spider diagram, write a sentence to explain why this change/continuity occurred.
3. How much had treatment changed by c1900? Write a paragraph to explain the extent of change that occurred by this point.

Improvements in hospitals and the influence of Florence Nightingale

Hospitals in the 18th century

As we discovered in Chapter 2, most of England's hospitals had closed down when Henry VIII dissolved the monasteries in the 1530s. By 1700, there were only five hospitals left in the country – and they were all in London. The country did not invest in new hospitals.

However, new hospitals did begin to appear in other cities in the 18th century, founded using donations from wealthy people and from members of the new middle classes, such as lawyers and businessmen. Some doctors offered their services free of charge to these new hospitals so that they could practise their skills.

Attitudes towards the role of hospitals were changing, too. Hospitals increasingly became places where sick people were treated, as opposed to places where people could rest and pray. Doctors visited patients regularly and there was a surgeon or apothecary on site for daily treatments. A small staff of untrained nurses cared for the patients.

However, hospitals were still not places that people often chose to be treated. The rich received medical treatment, and even surgery, in their own homes, which was much safer.

Hospitals were still quite particular about who they treated. Generally, patients admitted were 'the deserving poor' – respectable, working class people who could not afford to pay their medical bills. This change in the types of people hospitals were willing to treat was very important in the history of medical treatment, because it gave poor people access to trained doctors for the first time.

Unfortunately, as more people started to attend, hospitals became less sanitary. They became less strict about turning away infectious patients.

Although they often had separate wards for infectious patients. However, doctors went from patient to patient and ward to ward without washing their hands or changing their clothes. Diseases spread quickly. People did not understand that germs caused disease, so they did not take steps to avoid spreading the germs.

By the middle of the 19th century, there were a lot more hospitals. However, hospital conditions were very poor.

Florence Nightingale

Source A

A photograph of Florence Nightingale, taken in 1855.

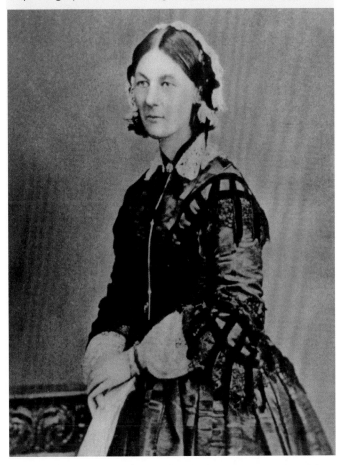

It was in these dirty hospital conditions that Florence Nightingale found herself when she began nursing. Nightingale was born into a wealthy family in 1820. When she was 17, she experienced a religious vision telling her that her mission was to serve mankind. She eventually convinced her parents to allow her to train as a nurse, first in Germany and then in Paris. In 1853, she became the superintendent of nurses at King's College Hospital in London.

In 1854, Britain went to war with Russia in the Crimea. News reports said that the hospitals there were not fit for the soldiers to be treated in, and there was a national outcry at the rumours that there were no nurses or even bandages available to the soldiers. Because of this outcry, and her position in society, Nightingale was able to convince the government to send her to improve the hospitals in the Crimea, along with 38 other nurses.

While Nightingale was in the Crimea, she made changes to the care of the wounded soldiers in many different ways.

- Nightingale and her nurses demanded 300 scrubbing brushes to get rid of any dirt near patients being treated.
- Nurses were organised to treat nearly 2,000 wounded soldiers.
- Clean bedding and good meals were provided.

Nightingale's efforts had a very positive effect on the mortality rate – within six months, it had dropped from 40% to only 2%.

By the time Nightingale returned to Britain in 1856, she was a national hero. There had been a great deal of bad publicity about the conditions in war hospitals, and Nightingale was famous for having made a big difference. This gave her credibility and helped her to make changes to hospitals in Britain, too.

Extend your knowledge

Statistics

Florence Nightingale was also one of the first people to use statistical diagrams to persuade people that there was a need for change. One of her diagrams was called 'Cause of Mortality in the Army in the East'.

Source B

A copy of a ballad that was written about Nightingale in 1855. Ballads like this, set to popular tunes from the time, would sell for a penny on street corners.

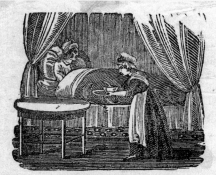

The Nightingale In the East.

TUNE,—"THE COTTAGE AND WATER MILL."

Ryle & Co., Printers, 2 & 3, Monmouth Court, Seven Dials. London.

ON a dark lonely night on the Crimea's dread
    shore,
There had been bloodshed and strife on the morn-
    ing before,
The dead and the dying lay bleeding around,
Some crying for help—there was none to be found
Now God in his mercy he pity'd their cries,
And the soldier so cheerful in the morning doth rise
So forward my lads, may your heart never fail,
You are cheer'd by the presence of a sweet
    Nightingale.

Now God sent this woman to succour the brave,
Some thousands she's say'd from an untimely grave
Her eyes beam with pleasure, she's bounteous
    and good,
The wants of the wounded are by her understood
With fever some brought in, with life almost gone
Some with dismantled limbs, some to fragments
    is torn,
But they keep up their spirits, their hearts never fail
Now they're cheer'd by the presence of a sweet
    Nightingale.

Her heart it means good—for no bounty she'll take
She'd lay down her life for the poor soldier's sake
She prays for the dying, she gives peace to the
    brave,
She feels that a soldier has a soul to be saved.
The wounded they love her, as it has been seen,
She's the soldier's preserver, they call her their
    queen,
May God give her strength, & her heart never fail,
One of Heaven's best gifts is Miss Nightingale.

The wives of the wounded how thankful are they,
Their husbands are car'd for, how happy are they.
Whate'er her country, this gift God has given.
The soldiers they say she's an angel from Heaven
Sing praise to this woman, and deny it who can !
And all women was sent for the comfort of man,
Let's hope no more against them you'll rail,
Treat them well, and they'll prove like Miss
    Nightingale.

Source C

In this extract from *Notes on Hospitals*, published in 1859, Nightingale explains how important it is for hospitals to be well-ventilated.

To build a hospital with one closed court with high walls, or what is worse, with two closed courts, is to stagnate the air even before it reaches the wards.

This defect is one of the most serious that can be committed in hospital architecture; and it exists, nevertheless, in some form or other in nearly all the older hospitals, and in many even of recent constructions.

The air outside the hospital cannot be maintained in a state sufficiently pure to be used for internal ventilation, unless there be entire freedom of movement. Anything which interferes with this is injurious. Neighbouring high walls, smoking chimneys, trees, high ground, are all more or less hurtful; but worse than all is bad construction of the hospital itself.

The impact of Florence Nightingale in British hospitals

Following her return from the Crimea, Nightingale's experience and popularity meant that she was able to have a big impact on hospital care in Britain in two different ways: **the way hospitals were designed** and **the training of nurses**.

For example, Nightingale preferred hospitals to follow the pavilion plan. This meant they were built with improved ventilation, with more windows, larger rooms and separate isolation wards to stop diseases spreading (see Source D).

Also, Nightingale established a nursing school at St Thomas' Hospital in London called the Nightingale School for Nurses in 1860. Figure 3.5 gives more detail on the impact of Nightingale's work.

Extend your knowledge

Nursing now

Now known as the Florence Nightingale Faculty of Nursing and Midwifery, Nightingale's school has been connected to St Thomas' Hospital ever since it was founded by Nightingale in 1860.

I wrote *Notes on Nursing* in 1859, setting out the key role of a nurse and the importance of thorough training.

In 1860, I set up the Nightingale School for Nurses at St Thomas' Hospital, London. Here, nurses were trained mainly on sanitary matters.

On my recommendations, new hospitals were built out of materials that could be easily cleaned. I believe dirt spreads disease, so tiles on the floors and painted walls and ceilings made it possible to wash down all surfaces and get rid of this dirt.

I made nursing seem like a respectable occupation. 'Nightingale nurses' were more often middle-class women. Previously, nurses had been from working-class backgrounds, and had a reputation for being drunk, flirtatious and uncaring.

I promoted 'pavilion style' hospitals, where separate wards were built in hospitals to ensure infectious patients could be kept separate.

Rigorous training turned nursing into a profession, rather than a simple, unskilled job. This encouraged more women to sign up, and so the number and skill of nurses grew rapidly.

Figure 3.5 The impact of Florence Nightingale's work.

Hospitals by 1900

Hospitals by 1900 looked very different from the few in Britain in 1700. Many different wards split up infectious patients from those requiring surgery. Operating theatres and specialist departments for new medical equipment provided separate spaces for certain procedures.

Cleanliness was now of the utmost importance: hospitals first focused on cleaning up germs using **antiseptics**, and by 1900 they were focused on preventing the germs from getting in to begin with. Doctors were a common sight, particularly junior doctors who were training and getting more hands-on experience. Trained nurses lived in nearby houses provided for them.

New ideas about hospitals were adopted quickly. Everybody wanted to have the most modern hospital designs, to help them attract donations and new student doctors.

The function of hospitals had completely changed. Instead of being places for the sick to rest, hospitals had become a place where the sick were treated. This fundamental change in the role of hospitals had forced a change in the way they were built and run.

Source D

This picture and plan show the Birmingham hospital that was opened in 1888. It was built on open ground with separate isolation wards, modelled on the pavilion plan favoured by Florence Nightingale.

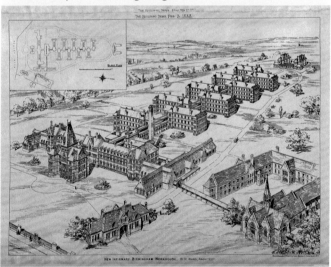

Activities ?

1 List the changes that had occurred in hospitals by c1900.

2 Explain the impact of more people attending hospitals.

3 Write an obituary for Florence Nightingale, explaining the impact she had on nursing and hospital design.

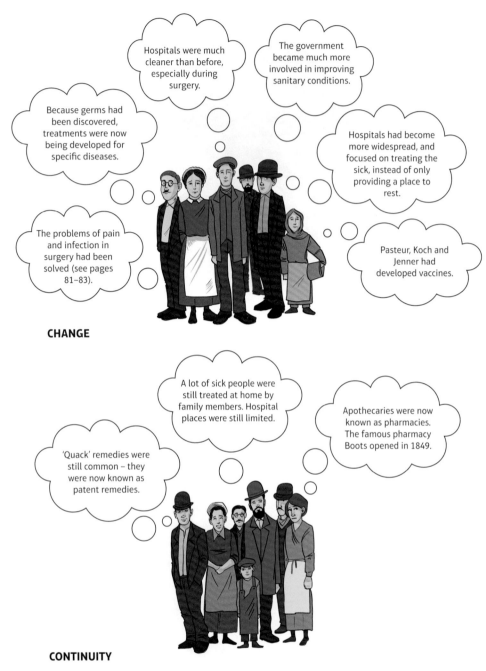

CHANGE

CONTINUITY

Figure 3.6 Extent of change in care and treatment.

Improvements in surgical treatment

In the 18th century, surgery was a dangerous and usually fatal business. The three big problems that surgeons faced were:

- bleeding
- pain
- infection.

Although substances like opium had been used for some time to calm patients with severe injuries, without **anaesthetic** there was no way of preventing the excruciating pain that they went through – which sometimes sent them into shock. Surgeries had to be performed quickly, before the patient bled to death on the operating table, as blood transfusions had not yet been developed. **Bleeding** continued to be a problem during surgery throughout the 18th and 19th centuries.

The most talented surgeons were able to operate extremely quickly, which improved their patients' chances of survival. However, even if the patient survived, often infection set in as surgeries were not performed in germ-free environments. In fact, they were usually performed in the patient's home, with the surgeon wearing the same clothes he had arrived in.

For these reasons, surgical treatments were quite limited. The most common type of surgery was amputation, which was often necessary due to accidents or complications relating to tuberculosis. Other types of surgeries were rare because the danger of death was so great. However, surgeons were becoming more respected.

In the 19th century, significant developments occurred that tackled two of the three problems of surgery. Firstly, anaesthetics were developed to enable surgeons to put patients to sleep before operating on them – which helped with the **pain**. Secondly, the development of Germ Theory led to an understanding of the importance of cleanliness in the operating room, and **antiseptic surgery** was developed – this helped to stop **infection**.

Tackling pain: the development of the anaesthetic

Doctors had been experimenting with pain relief for their patients for many centuries, in an attempt to keep them still and quiet for long enough to perform operations. Early experiments with laughing gas proved quite successful for small operations such as pulling teeth. When the chemical ether was discovered and used in America, it caused great excitement among surgeons. However, there were some problems with ether. It often made patients vomit, and the gas irritated the lungs which caused coughing, even while the patient was unconscious. Worse still, it was very flammable, which meant it was a dangerous chemical to keep around, given that operating rooms were lit with candles or gas lamps.

James Simpson and chloroform

James Simpson, a young surgeon from Edinburgh, was convinced that there were better anaesthetics than laughing gas to be discovered. He gathered a group of friends together and they inhaled the vapours of

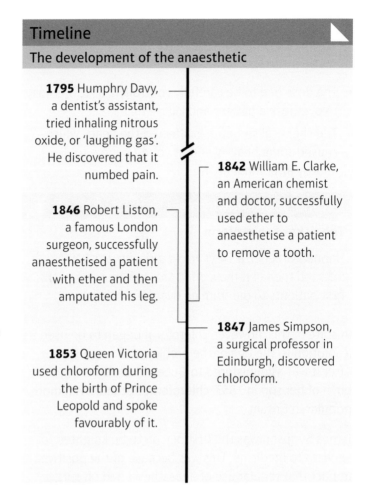

Timeline

The development of the anaesthetic

1795 Humphry Davy, a dentist's assistant, tried inhaling nitrous oxide, or 'laughing gas'. He discovered that it numbed pain.

1842 William E. Clarke, an American chemist and doctor, successfully used ether to anaesthetise a patient to remove a tooth.

1846 Robert Liston, a famous London surgeon, successfully anaesthetised a patient with ether and then amputated his leg.

1847 James Simpson, a surgical professor in Edinburgh, discovered chloroform.

1853 Queen Victoria used chloroform during the birth of Prince Leopold and spoke favourably of it.

various chemicals to see what might work. After sniffing chloroform, the entire party passed out and were discovered some time later by Mrs Simpson. Clearly, chloroform was an effective anaesthetic.

Source E

An artist's impression of the night when James Simpson and his friends discovered the power of chloroform, c1860.

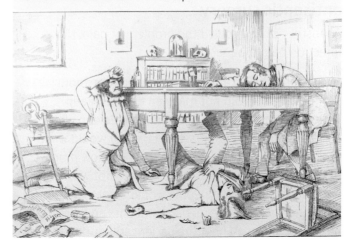

Although they weren't detected during Simpson's experiments, chloroform did have some negative side effects.

- The dose had to be carefully controlled, as it was easy to overdose a patient and kill them.
- The chemical sometimes affected the heart, which caused some healthy and fit young people to die shortly after inhaling it.

Extend your knowledge

The risks of chloroform

Hannah Greener, a 14-year-old girl who was having an infected toenail removed in 1848, became one of the first patients to die from an overdose of chloroform.

In spite of this, however, chloroform began to be used as a solution to the one of the problems of surgery: pain. After it was administered to Queen Victoria during the birth of her son in 1853, chloroform became even more popular in Britain.

James Simpson was the first person to be knighted for services to medicine. This was because of the positive impact that regular use of anaesthesia had on surgery. More surgeries took place and deeper, more complex surgeries became possible.

Some historians suggest that the use of anaesthetics made it possible for doctors to attempt lengthier and more-complex operations. However, because anaesthetics allowed for deeper surgery to be attempted, infection and bleeding became even bigger problems.

Tackling infection: the development of antiseptic surgery

Anaesthetics had solved the problem of pain. Now, infection had to be tackled.

Historically, due to a lack of understanding about germs, surgeons did not make an effort to keep their surroundings, or even themselves, clean when they operated on patients. In fact, many would wear their most stained doctor's coat to show how much experience they had. Instruments were not washed, and a large number of people would be present during operations – including medical students and 'dressers', whose job it was to hold the patient still during the operation. As a result of this, many patients survived operations but then died shortly afterwards from infections such as gangrene or sepsis.

Joseph Lister and carbolic acid

Joseph Lister was an English surgeon. By studying infected wounds, he realised that the flesh was rotting. Lister compared his results with the recently-published work of Pasteur, who had identified germs as being responsible for decay. Lister theorised that, if microbes in the air caused wine and vinegar to go bad, perhaps microbes also caused flesh to rot.

Lister started to look for a chemical that would clear bacteria from wounds. He was aware of the use of carbolic acid in sewage treatments. So, in 1865, he operated on a patient with a broken leg and added a bandage soaked in carbolic acid. The wound healed cleanly.

From this, Lister developed a series of steps to ensure that wounds did not become infected. These included spraying **carbolic acid** in the air during operations.

Source F

This famous picture is taken from William Watson Cheyne's book *Antiseptic Surgery* which was published in 1882.

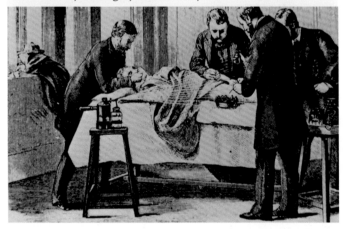

Lister published his results in *The Lancet*, a medical journal. He detailed 11 different cases where carbolic acid had been used successfully in surgery.

In spite of its success, antiseptic surgery did not catch on quickly.

- News of Lister's success spread more quickly than Germ Theory. However, this meant that the science behind the new method wasn't fully understood. Consequently, not all surgeons were willing to use the carbolic spray. They still did not believe that the air was full of germs.

- Carbolic spray dried out the skin and left behind an odd smell. Some surgeons argued that, since it made their hands sore, it certainly could not be doing the patient any good.
- Lister focused on encouraging his colleagues to use the carbolic spray instead of scientifically proving his theory. He was a 'doer' rather than a 'thinker'.

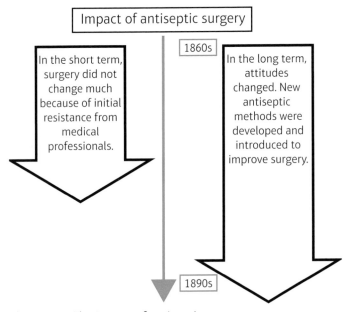

Figure 3.7 The impact of antiseptic surgery.

The key change here wasn't that doctors started using carbolic acid – although it was a great improvement, carbolic spray was only popular for a short amount of time, and even Lister himself stopped using it in 1890. What is important is that the attitude of surgeons towards antiseptic and aseptic surgery* changed. Surgeons finally understood that performing safe surgery was not only possible – it was their duty.

Key term

Aseptic surgery*

Surgery where microbes are prevented from getting into a wound in the first place, as opposed to being killed off with an antiseptic.

Other surgeons began to look for different methods of preventing infection. By 1900, instruments were steam cleaned, operating theatres were scrubbed spotless, rubber gloves and surgical gowns were introduced and surgeons used face masks during operations.

Opposition to change

Although developments in anaesthetics and antiseptics helped to improve the effectiveness and availability of surgery, not everybody welcomed the changes.

- Anaesthetics allowed for deeper surgeries to be attempted. Before the introduction of carbolic spray, infection and bleeding became even bigger problems. The death rate actually increased, which seemed to suggest that anaesthetics were bad. People did not trust the technique.
- The Victorians believed that pain relief was interfering with God's plan, particularly in childbirth, which was meant to be painful.
- Some doctors believed that patients were more likely to die if they were unconscious during the operation, rather than awake and screaming.
- It took a long time for doctors to accept that germs caused infection. Surgeons did not want to believe that they might have been responsible for the infections that killed their patients.

Activities

1. Create an annotated timeline to show the changes that took place in the field of surgery during the 19th century.
2. Make flashcards for Simpson and Lister, explaining what they did and what impact this had on surgical techniques.
3. Have a debate with a partner about which key individual had the biggest impact. Use the flashcards you made to help you.

Exam-style question, Section B

Explain why there was rapid change in surgical treatments in the period c1700–c1900.

You may use the following in your answer:

- chloroform
- Joseph Lister.

You **must** also use information of your own. **12 marks**

Exam tip

Make sure that you focus on the reasons why development of surgical treatment was rapid – avoid simply describing the use of anaesthetics and antiseptics.

Case study – Jenner and the development of the vaccination

Smallpox in 18th-century Britain

At the start of this period, smallpox was a terrible threat to the health of the population of Britain. There were nationwide epidemics in 1722, 1723 and 1740–42. The problem was particularly bad in London, where there were 11 epidemics in the 18th century. The worst of these occurred in 1796, when 3,548 people died. By this time, the population of the city was approaching one million, so the disease spread quickly and easily from person to person.

At this time, people were still unaware of the cause of the disease, but they did have some ideas about how to avoid catching it. It had been noticed that people who caught a mild form of smallpox and then recovered from it did not catch it again. This would later form the basis for vaccination, which works in the same way. However, in the 18th century there was not enough scientific knowledge for people to understand how this worked.

Therefore, some people attempted to inoculate* themselves against smallpox by catching a mild dose of the disease, so that they would avoid catching a more severe form of it later on. Pus from a smallpox scab would be rubbed into a cut on the patient being inoculated by a doctor. Unfortunately, this did not always work: some patients died of the smallpox they were given, as the disease did not affect everyone in the same way.

Key term

Inoculate*
Deliberately infecting oneself with a disease, in order to avoid a more severe case of it later on.

In spite of this, inoculation was seen by many as the best chance of surviving smallpox. However, the procedure was very expensive and so only the very rich could afford it. Many doctors made a fortune carrying out inoculations for wealthy people. One doctor, Thomas Dimsdale, was made a baron, paid £10,000 and awarded an annual salary of £500 after he inoculated Catherine the Great and her children in 1768. He was one of the most successful **inoculators** of his time.

Jenner discovers the vaccination for smallpox

Edward Jenner was a Gloucestershire doctor in the late 18th century. He had trained as an apprentice to a surgeon-apothecary and then practised medicine at St George's Hospital in London, before returning to Gloucestershire, where he became a general practitioner (GP). Jenner was particularly interested in inoculations. He gathered evidence of over 1,000 cases where smallpox inoculation had failed.

There were a lot of dairy farms in the area where Jenner worked. He regularly treated dairy maids for cowpox* and noticed that, when there was a smallpox epidemic, those who had previously suffered from cowpox did not catch smallpox. He decided the two must be somehow connected.

Key term

Cowpox*
A disease causing red blisters on the skin, similar to smallpox. It can be transmitted from cows to humans.

Jenner needed to test his theory and so, in 1796, he infected a local boy, James Phipps, with cowpox. Six weeks later he attempted to infect James with smallpox, but James did not catch it. Jenner infected more local people with cowpox to further test his theory. In 1798, he wrote up his findings in *An Enquiry into the Causes and Effects of the Variola Vaccinae*. He named the technique 'vaccination' after the Latin word for cow, *vacca*.

Jenner made sure that the instructions for his new method were very detailed, so that other doctors would be able to follow them. He wanted other people to use the vaccination to prevent smallpox from spreading.

Reactions to the new vaccination

As with so many medical discoveries, it took some time for people to accept vaccinations. Although Jenner knew that the system worked, he was not able to explain how or why it worked – and this made people suspicious. The idea of infecting someone with an animal disease was seen as extremely strange, and a lot of people were against it.

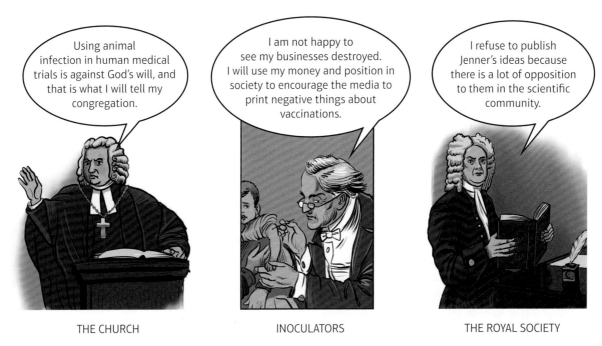

THE CHURCH INOCULATORS THE ROYAL SOCIETY

Figure 3.8 Differing opinions about vaccinations in the 19th century.

Although certain groups of people were against vaccinations, there was another, very powerful group that were in favour of them: parliament. As you can see from the timeline below, the British government favoured the new method of vaccination from the first half of the 19th century. This was because it was a safer and more reliable alternative to inoculation. It was also cheaper, because recipients of vaccines did not need to be put into quarantine, whereas those receiving the inoculation were in danger of spreading smallpox to other people.

> ### Key term
>
> **Public Vaccinators***
>
> Doctors paid by the government to vaccinate people against smallpox.

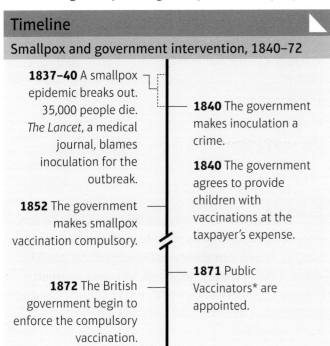

Timeline

Smallpox and government intervention, 1840–72

1837–40 A smallpox epidemic breaks out. 35,000 people die. *The Lancet*, a medical journal, blames inoculation for the outbreak.

1852 The government makes smallpox vaccination compulsory.

1872 The British government begin to enforce the compulsory vaccination.

1840 The government makes inoculation a crime.

1840 The government agrees to provide children with vaccinations at the taxpayer's expense.

1871 Public Vaccinators* are appointed.

> **Key individual: Edward Jenner**
> Jenner was a trained doctor who had worked as a surgeon and apothecary as well as in a hospital. He used careful scientific method to test and prove his vaccination.

> **Key institution: Government**
> The British government played an important role in promoting the vaccine. They provided funding and set up a society to promote vaccination. Later, they made it compulsory for everybody.

SMALLPOX VACCINATION

> **Observation and experimentation**
> Jenner observed the pattern of cowpox and smallpox in dairy maids. He planned his experiment carefully and then repeated it several times so that he could be certain it had not been just a fluke.

Figure 3.9 Factors assisting Jenner in developing the smallpox vaccine.

Activity ?

Create a six-picture storyboard to show how Edward Jenner developed the smallpox vaccine.

The impact of the smallpox vaccine

Short term

In the short term, the smallpox vaccine saved many lives. It quickly became very popular overseas and by 1800, 100,000 people around the world had been vaccinated. The French commander Napoleon had his entire army vaccinated in 1805.

The vaccination was slower to become popular in Britain, thanks to the anti-Jenner propaganda promoted by inoculators. Sometimes people still contracted smallpox or died of infection, because the doctors carrying out the procedure mixed up smallpox and cowpox samples or reused needles, and this discouraged people as well. However, after the Royal Jennerian Society had been founded in 1803, 12,000 British people were vaccinated in the space of two years.

Source G

This cartoon was drawn by Cruikshank in 1812. It is titled, '*The cowpox tragedy: scene the last.*' The year before, people vaccinated with cowpox had developed smallpox, because of an error with the samples used.

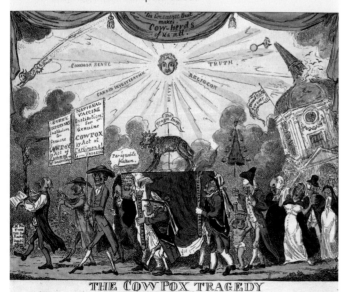

THE COWPOX TRAGEDY
— Scene the Last. —

Long term

By the end of the 19th century, vaccination against smallpox had become normal. Opposition continued throughout the century, but the number of people saved made it clear that the method worked. The number of smallpox cases fell dramatically from 1872, when the government started to enforce compulsory vaccinations – this meant that everyone had to be vaccinated for smallpox.

Extend your knowledge

Smallpox today

In the very long term, it could be argued that Jenner was responsible for the end of smallpox. In 1979, The World Health Organisation announced that the disease had been completely wiped out. This would not have been possible without Jenner's early work.

Jenner had shown that a vaccine could be used to stop smallpox from spreading. His work inspired other scientists, like Pasteur and Koch, to search for vaccinations for other diseases. However, there were no other vaccinations discovered that worked in the same way as the smallpox vaccine. This was a one-off, so scientists were unable to develop other vaccines based on Jenner's method.

Exam-style question, Section B

Explain why there was rapid change in the prevention of smallpox after 1798.

You may use the following information in your answer:

- inoculation
- the government.

You **must** also use information of your own.

12 marks

Exam tip

As well as explaining medical breakthroughs in your answer, in order to show what changed you should compare with the situation before Jenner's research.

New approaches to prevention: the development and use of vaccinations

People still generally believed that the best way to avoid dying from a disease was not catching it at all. People had begun to have new ideas about cures – however, most of these were still not effective on patients who were suffering from a disease. Therefore, scientists continued to focus on prevention and developed the idea of the **vaccination**.

Pasteur presented his case for the germ theory of infection in 1878, after publishing his Germ Theory in 1861. He theorised that microorganisms were responsible for disease. He admired the work of Jenner and started to look for vaccines that would tackle lots of diseases. However, Jenner's work had been the result of observations and experiments, rather than tackling the specific microbe. It would not be possible for other vaccines to work the same way. Pasteur realised that vaccines could only be developed once the germs causing that specific disease had been identified.

Pasteur's first effort at a vaccine was for **chicken cholera**. He identified the germ causing the disease and set about developing a vaccination against it.

In 1879 Pasteur proved that a weakened strain of the disease worked to vaccinate the chickens. He continued with his work, also creating a vaccine for anthrax, another devastating disease affecting animals. He then developed a vaccine for rabies.

Pasteur's work on vaccines involved producing a weakened version of the culture and then treating patients with it. This created an **immune response**, where the body fought off the weakened disease and, in doing so, created antibodies* that prevented the individual from suffering from that disease if the microorganism was encountered again. Pasteur did not know that this was why the vaccine worked, because science had not progressed far enough for him to investigate the method properly yet. However, his methods were clearly effective.

Key term

Antibodies*

Particles inside the body that identify and help to remove germs. The body creates them when first encounters the germ, so that it can fight off the same disease more easily if it comes back.

Until this point, Pasteur's focus had been on animal diseases that caused problems for farmers. His work on vaccinations had little direct impact on disease in humans. However, it inspired research among other scientists, who wanted to find other vaccines for a wide range of human diseases.

Koch's work isolating the microbes that caused specific diseases (see page 71) was very important in developing new vaccines. For example, in 1890, Emil von Behring developed a vaccine against tetanus and diphtheria.

By 1900, scientists all over the world were busy isolating microbes and developing vaccines, thanks to the work of Pasteur and Koch. This was a significant breakthrough in the **prevention** of disease.

Activities ❓

1 Draw a storyboard to explain how vaccines were developed.

2 As a method of prevention, vaccines were more effective than anything that had been tried in previous centuries. What factors made the development of new vaccinations possible?

The Public Health Act, 1875

Alongside the new scientific methods of prevention, a great deal was also being done to improve living conditions in Britain, particularly in the larger cities. In c1700, the government had little interest in improving conditions in cities. They had a *laissez-faire** attitude and believed that it was not their responsibility or right to interfere in the way that people lived.

Key word

*Laissez-faire**

This French term means 'leave be'. It is used to describe governments who do not get involved in the day-to-day lives of their population.

During the 1800s, this attitude began to change. More men now had the right to vote, so the government began passing laws that appealed to the masses. The government knew that if they appealed to normal people, they would be voted into power in future elections.

As well as this, cholera arrived in Britain. The epidemic led to the deaths of thousands of people. The work of John Snow (see page 92) led people to believe that cholera was spread in dirty water, and this theory was backed up by Pasteur's discovery of microorganisms in 1861.

Extend your knowledge

Edwin Chadwick

In 1842, Edwin Chadwick published his *Report on the Sanitary Conditions of the Labouring Classes*. He had spent some time researching among the urban poor, and this book detailed the results of his research. He showed that people living in cities had a much lower life expectancy than people living in the countryside.

Chadwick concluded that this was down to the filthy living conditions in cities. He campaigned for all cities to set up boards of health, who would be responsible for supplying clean water and disposing of sewage.

Chadwick's work did not have much impact on conditions at the time, but it was only one piece of the puzzle. After more evidence emerged, supporting the theory that clean water was vital for a healthy population, the government was more willing to act.

From the 1860s, the government began to take more action to improve living conditions for people in cities.

- In London, 1,300 miles of sewers were built by 1865.
- In Birmingham, slums were demolished.
- In Leeds, a local business obtained a court order to prevent sewage from being drained into the river from which they got their water.

There had been a change in the way people felt about public health. More people began to recognise that it was now everybody's responsibility.

Extend your knowledge

The first Public Health Act, 1848

The aim of the first Public Health Act was to improve the sanitary condition of towns in England and Wales by encouraging cities to set up boards of health and provide clean water supplies. However, it was not compulsory, so did not have much impact on the health of the people. It was not until 1875 that rules were put in place to improve sanitary conditions that were compulsory – they had to be followed.

Developments in understanding…	Factors, c1700–c1900	Factor
CAUSE	• Germ theory. • The development of work on **identifying microbes**.	• Role of technology (microscopes). • Role of science of chemistry. • Role of individuals.
TREATMENT	• Better **hospitals** and **nursing** thanks to the work of Florence Nightingale. • Improvements in surgical treatment, because of **anaesthetics** and **antiseptic surgery**.	• Role of individuals. • Role of science of chemistry.
PREVENTION	• Development of **vaccinations** begun by Edward Jenner. • **Improved water supply and drainage**, with two Public Health Acts in 1848 and 1875.	• Role of individuals. • Role of government.

In response to this change in attitude, the government passed the **second Public Health Act** in 1875.

City authorities had to follow the rules it set out. The responsibilities included:

- providing clean water to stop diseases that were spread in dirty water
- disposing of sewage to prevent drinking and washing water from becoming polluted
- building public toilets to avoid pollution
- employing a public officer of health to monitor outbreaks of diseases
- ensuring new houses were of better quality, to stop damp and overcrowding

- providing public parks for exercise
- inspecting lodging houses to make sure they were clean and healthy
- creating street lighting to prevent accidents
- checking the quality of the food in shops to make sure that it didn't contain anything that could cause somebody harm. For example, some bakers mixed chalk into flour to make bread whiter.

The government had taken solid steps to prevent the spread of disease – and it worked. The last cholera epidemic in Britain was in 1866–67, and it had a lower mortality rate than previous epidemics, due to some of the new measures that had been put in place.

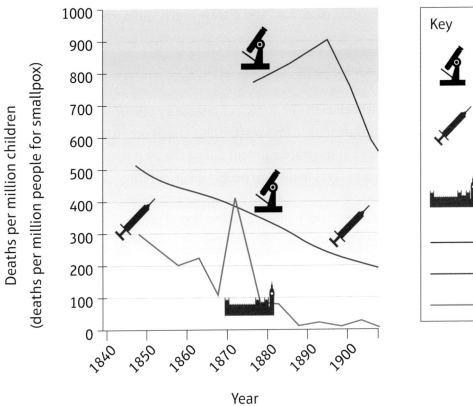
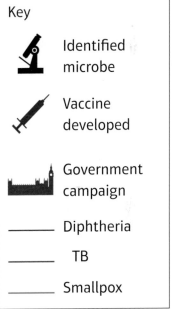

Figure 3.10 Mortality rates of major diseases, 1840–1900.

Summary

- By c1900, the treatment and prevention of disease had changed. This was due to an improved understanding of the cause of disease.
- More hospitals were built, making treatments more widely available.
- Hospitals were cleaner and built to provide a space for recovery, thanks to the work of Florence Nightingale. Nursing had become a respectable profession.
- Herbal and patent remedies were still popular for common illnesses, because few new treatments had been developed.
- Surgical procedures had become a more effective method of treatment as a result of the development of anaesthetics and antiseptics. However, blood loss was still a problem, so surgeons still had to work quickly.
- Scientists had developed a method for vaccinating people against diseases and had begun to develop vaccines for particular illnesses.
- One of these illnesses was smallpox – Edward Jenner proved that catching cowpox prevented people from catching smallpox.
- In the 19th century, the government began to take action to improve public health in cities. This was a result of a better understanding of the link between dirty conditions and disease and it led to a healthier population.

Checkpoint

Strengthen

S1 What changes and continuities had there been in the treatment of disease by c1900?

S2 Describe the actions that Florence Nightingale took to improve hospital conditions in Britain.

S3 Identify the steps that led to improvements in surgical treatment during the 19th century.

S4 Create a flow diagram to show the different stages in the way people dealt with smallpox, in the period c1700–c1900.

S5 What were the short-term and long-term impacts of Jenner's new method of preventing smallpox?

Challenge

C1 As in the previous period (c1500–c1700), attitudes in society had a big impact on change in treatment. Can you list three ways that people's attitudes encouraged developments in treatment and prevention, and three ways that they held them back?

C2 Compare this list to the one you made at the end of Section 2.2. Had people's attitudes changed or stayed the same between these two periods? Explain your answer, using examples from the text where possible.

If you are not confident about any of these questions, form a group with other students, discuss the answers and then record your conclusions. Your teacher can give you some hints.

Learning outcomes

- Understand how the government tackled the cholera epidemics of the 19th century.

Source A

This cartoon was drawn in 1852, for the magazine *Punch*.

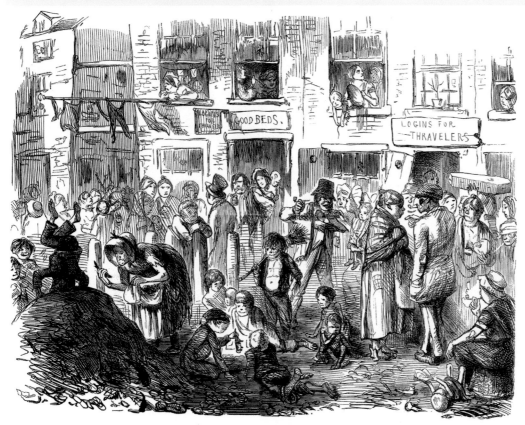

A COURT FOR KING CHOLERA.

Fighting cholera

Cholera was a terrible disease. It caused diarrhoea and sickness that became so bad, the victim would become dehydrated*. It was usually fatal: sufferers would die between two and six days after falling sick. As the sufferer became dehydrated, their blood would become thicker, rupturing blood vessels under the skin. This turned the skin blue, so cholera was nicknamed 'the blue death'. It was spread through person-to-person contact, or water contaminated with the faeces of a sufferer.

Cholera did not arrive in Britain until 1831. It spread quickly across the country. It arrived in London in February 1832 and there were 5,275 deaths in the city by the end of the year. Cholera mainly affected the poorest people. There were lots of cases in slum dwellings, as well as in workhouses, prisons and asylums. However, wealthier districts were not immune. As had been the case with the plague two centuries earlier, doctors found it impossible to treat. There were three further severe epidemics across the country in the following decades.

Key term

Dehydrated*
When the body does not have enough water to keep the organs working properly.

Activity ?

Look carefully at the cartoon. List all the threats to health you can see in the picture.

Year of epidemic	Total cholera-related deaths in England and Wales
1831–32	21,882
1848–49	53,293
1853–54	20,097
1865–66	14,378

Attempts to prevent the spread of cholera

Some steps were taken to try to clean up the filthiest areas of the cities and so prevent the spread of cholera. The belief that miasmata and rotting material caused disease was still widespread, so local councils and populations turned their attentions to the mess in which they were living. The government encouraged cities to set up boards of health and provide clean water supplies. However, this did not have a great effect on people's living conditions.

Source B

This letter was printed in *The Times* in 1849, during the second cholera outbreak. It was written by a group of residents of Soho, London.

Sir, May we be and beseech your protection and power. We are Sir, as it may be, living in a wilderness, so far as the rest of London knows anything of us, or as the rich and great people care about. We live in muck and filth. We ain't got no privies [toilets], no dust bins, no drains, no water-supplies, and no drain or sewer in the whole place. The Sewer Company, in Greek Street, Soho Square, all great, rich powerful men take no notice whatsoever of our complaints. The stench of a gully-hole is disgusting. We all of us suffer, and numbers are ill, and if the cholera comes Lord help us all.

John Snow

John Snow was a surgeon who had moved to Soho in 1836 and had become London's leading anaesthetist. It was Snow who gave Queen Victoria chloroform during the birth of Prince Leopold in 1851. He was popular and well-respected.

Source C

This cartoon was published in *Punch* in 1858. In it, the River Thames is offering his 'children' to London – the diseases diphtheria, scrofula (a type of tuberculosis) and cholera.

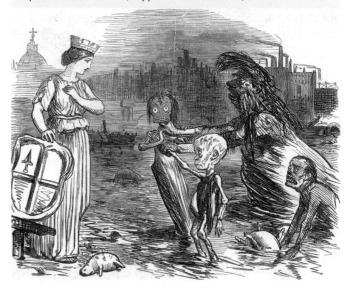

Snow observed cholera during the epidemic of 1848–49. He wrote up his theories in *On the Mode of Communication of Cholera*. In it, he suggested that:

- cholera could not be transmitted by a miasma, because it affected the guts, not the lungs
- drinking water was being contaminated by the cholera-ridden faeces being disposed of in the city's drains.

Snow concluded that cholera was transmitted by dirty drinking water.

The 1854 epidemic

In August of 1854, cholera broke out in Soho, where Snow lived. This prompted Snow to investigate the 93 deaths in his local area.

Snow created a spot map to show where the deaths had occurred in the area around Golden Square and Broad Street. He took a street map and drew spots onto it to represent the deaths that had taken place (see Source D).

Source D

A section of John Snow's cholera spot map, 1854.

After looking at the map, John Snow realised that there was a pattern: the number of deaths seemed to be centred around the water pump on Broad Street.

To Snow, it was clear that the water pump was the source of the infection. He removed the handle from the pump, preventing locals from pumping water, and the cholera outbreak went away as quickly as it had arrived.

Later inspections of the well underneath the water pump revealed that it was extremely close to a cesspit* – less than one metre away. Although the cesspit had a brick lining, it had cracked, meaning waste from the cesspit was seeping into the well and spreading cholera.

Key term

Cesspit*

A pit for storing sewage or waste.

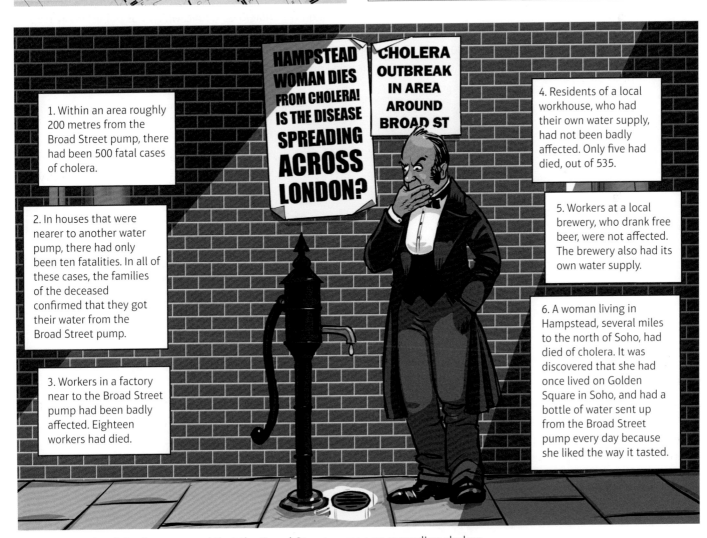

Figure 3.11 How John Snow proved that the Broad Street pump was spreading cholera.

The impact and significance of John Snow and the Broad Street pump

In 1855, Snow presented his findings to a House of Commons committee. He showed the evidence that he had gathered, which proved that cholera was transmitted by dirty water. He recommended that the government start making massive improvements in the sewer systems of London. By doing this, Snow argued, another cholera outbreak could be avoided.

The government did eventually agree to invest in a new sewer system, which was planned by Joseph Bazalgette and completed in 1875. However, this was not just due to the work of John Snow. An unusually hot and dry summer in 1858 had caused 'The Great Stink'. The Thames was low and the stench of the exposed sewage on the riverbanks heating up and steaming gently in the sun became terrible. This nudged the government into action and the work on the new sewers was begun in 1860.

Many people rejected Snow's work. Other scientists pointed out that cases would still occur among people who lived further away from the pump, even if they were drinking less of the water. The General Board of Health clung to the theory of miasma and rejected Snow's findings. Admitting that cholera was present in the water would mean having to take steps to provide clean water, which was going to be very costly – and, the Board argued, there was no scientific proof that it would work.

Source E

These two drawings accompanied the General Board of Health's report on the cholera epidemic, which was published in 1855. The Board had rejected Snow's theory that cholera was spread through water. Here, they attempt to prove their theory by offering two drawings of water magnified 200 times. On the left, a drawing of water taken from the Broad Street pump. On the right, a drawing of water from the New River Company, elsewhere in London.

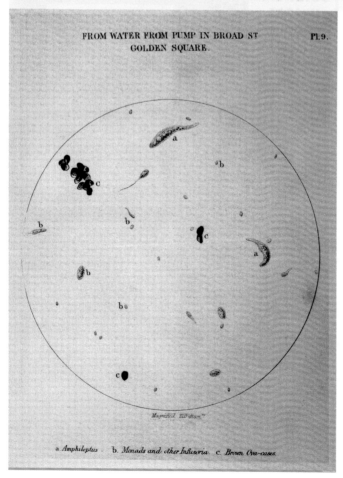

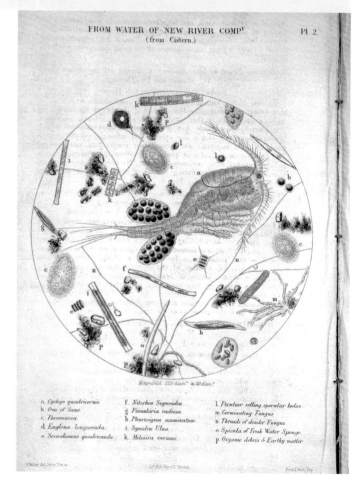

Although Snow had plenty of practical evidence to show that cholera was spread in water, he had no scientific evidence to show what caused the disease. It would be another seven years before Pasteur published his Germ Theory – three years after Snow had died – and another 30 years before Koch finally isolated the bacterium that caused the disease.

Therefore, in the short term, Snow's work had an immediate impact on the residents of Soho Square, many of whom avoided cholera thanks to his removal of the pump handle. However, his impact outside of this area was very limited. It was not until much later that the importance of clean water was accepted.

Preventing cholera: the role of individuals and institutions

Role of the government	Role of the individual: John Snow
Encouraged local councils to clean up their cities and provide clean water.	Observed the pattern of cholera cases.
Listened to John Snow's evidence about cholera.	Designed an experiment to prove that cholera was caused by dirty water.
Arranged for a new sewer system to be built in London.	Prevented residents from drinking the water.
Eventually passed the 1875 Public Health Act to force other cities to clean up.	Presented his findings to the government.

THINKING HISTORICALLY   Change and continuity (3b)

Significant to whom?

Historians are interested in different aspects of the past, and ask different questions. The interest of the historian is a very important factor in their decision about what is significant and what is not.

Historian's focus	Social historian	British historian	Scientific historian
Title of investigation	How did medical developments change living standards in Britain during the 19th century?	How did British scientists change our understanding of the causes of disease?	What role did science and technology play in the development of medicine?

Changes and events during the 19th century

In 1861, Pasteur identified that germs caused decay.	The British government passed laws to make cities cleaner and protect people's health.	In 1865, Lister developed a carbolic spray to make surgery safer.
In 1854, John Snow made a link between cholera and dirty water.	Better microscopes enabled scientists to see microbes and link them with diseases.	In 1797, Edward Jenner developed a vaccination against smallpox.
Robert Koch developed methods to allow bacteria to be grown and observed more easily.	The Enlightenment meant that people were more interested in looking for rational explanations for disease.	In 1870, John Tyndall theorised that dust particles carried germs that caused disease.

For each historian, make a diagram to show the relative significance of the changes and events that would interest them. Write the historian in the middle of the page and then add the events and changes that would interest them: the more significant, the closer to the historian.

1   Look at the change or event of most interest to the social historian. How important is it to the other historians?

2   Why would the work of Joseph Lister be of interest to the social historian and the scientific historian?

3   Would the British historian include the work of Pasteur or ignore it? Explain your answer.

4   How important is it for the reader to understand the interest and focus of the historian when reading their work?

Summary

- Cholera first appeared in Britain in 1831.
- There were four major epidemics in the 19th century and they particularly affected poor people living in cities.
- John Snow thought that cholera was spread by water, not by a miasma.
- During the 1854 epidemic, he mapped the cholera fatalities around Golden Square in Soho. The evidence suggested that the outbreak was connected to the Broad Street pump.
- Snow presented his findings to the government. However, they did not take action straight away.
- By 1858, the government were ready to take action to provide clean water for the population. The final outbreak of cholera was much less severe as a result of this action.

Checkpoint

Strengthen

S1 When were the four cholera epidemics in Britain?

S2 Describe the actions that John Snow took to prove that cholera was a water-borne disease.

S3 What event finally forced the British government to take action on cholera?

Challenge

C1 Explain why Snow's theory was not widely accepted when he published it.

C2 Attitudes in society were changing during this period and people were recognising the link between dirt and disease. How do the sources in this section show this?

If you are not confident about any of these questions, form a group with other students, discuss the answers and then record your conclusions. Your teacher can give you some hints.

Activity **?**

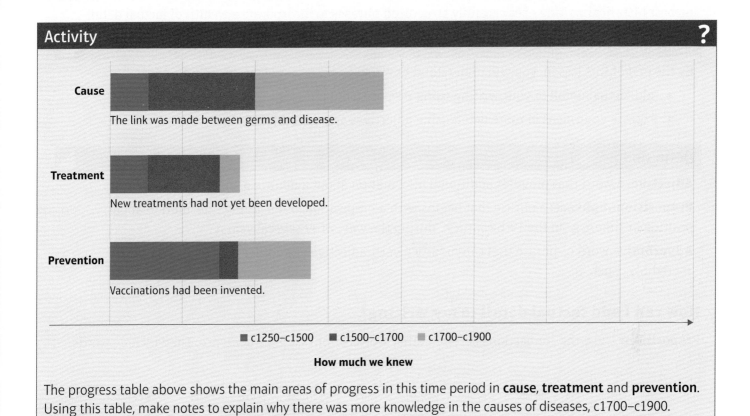

| | c1250–c1500 | c1500–c1700 | c1700–c1900 |

Cause
The link was made between germs and disease.

Treatment
New treatments had not yet been developed.

Prevention
Vaccinations had been invented.

How much we knew

The progress table above shows the main areas of progress in this time period in **cause**, **treatment** and **prevention**. Using this table, make notes to explain why there was more knowledge in the causes of diseases, c1700–c1900.

Recall quiz

1 Why did the search for rational explanations become more fashionable in the period c1700–c1900?

2 What theory had scientists come up with to explain disease in the early 18th century?

3 What was the impact of Pasteur's work?

4 Which disease-causing germs did Koch find when he was looking for microbes?

5 Why were herbal remedies still popular in the 19th century?

6 Where did Florence Nightingale test out her theories about the importance of clean hospitals?

7 Name two anaesthetics that were developed during this period.

8 List three points from the 1875 Public Health Act.

9 When did Jenner develop his vaccination against smallpox?

10 Where did John Snow trace the 1854 Soho cholera epidemic to?

Exam-style questions, Section B

'Louis Pasteur's publication of the Germ Theory was the biggest turning point in medicine in the period c1700-c1900'.

How far do you agree with this statement?

You may use the following information in your answer:

• Edward Jenner   • Robert Koch.

You **must** also use information of your own. **16 marks**

Exam tip

Remember to set out criteria against which to judge each turning point: did it have an impact on diagnosis, treatment, prevention, public health? Was the impact rapid or did it take time?

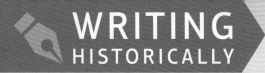

Writing historically: using phrases to build detail

The best historical writing uses carefully structured phrases to incorporate a wealth of factual detail.

Learning outcomes

By the end of this lesson, you will understand how to:

- add factual detail to your writing using prepositional phrases
- express your ideas in more detail using adjectives and adverbials.

Definitions

Adjective: a word that provides additional information about a noun, e.g. 'clear, precise writing'.

Prepositional phrase: a phrase that begins with a preposition, often giving information about position or time, e.g. 'in the 19th century', 'during the war', 'after several years'.

Adverbial: a word or phrase that can modify a verb, adjective or another adverb, e.g. 'quickly', 'incredibly', 'such'.

How can I add factual detail to my writing?

Prepositions show the connections between other words or phrases in a sentence. They include words like:

in	at	on	after	before	during	with	without	from	to	between

Prepositional phrases can be used to add important information about the time and/or place that significant events took place in. For example:

During the Crimean War...	In the early 1800s...	Before Pasteur's discovery...
With Koch's work on microbes...	Without this knowledge...	From 1853 to 1856...

1. Look at the response to this exam-style question. Rewrite the response, adding more information using prepositional phrases. The highlighted sections show where the answer needs more information – usually, **when** or **where** these events happened.

> 'The role of science and technology was the main reason why diagnosis improved in the 18th and 19th centuries'. How far do you agree? **(16 marks)**

The second part of the Scientific Revolution focused on finding answers to big questions in science. People wanted to prove new theories. Individuals helped improve diagnosis using science and technology. French chemist, Louis Pasteur, proved germ theory. Once this was known, the search for specific causes and specific treatments began. The breakthrough came with Robert Koch's work on microbes, identifying the germs that cause tuberculosis, was developed. Others followed, but all were dependent on the Pasteur's theory and being able to identify the individual causes. The British government rejected Germ Theory at first. Koch's visit to Calcutta was ignored.

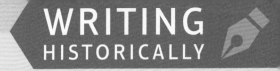
How can I add detail to my writing?

One way in which you can add more information to your answer is by adding **adjectives**, prepositional phrases and **adverbials**.

Compare these two versions of a sentence:

> *Florence Nightingale brought people new ideas. Without her experience in the war, the development of hospitals and training would not have benefitted people.*

> *Florence Nightingale brought the people of the United Kingdom new ideas on medical practice. Without her experience in the Crimean war, the development of clean hospitals and improved training of nurses would not have benefitted such a large number of people.*

Look at the copy of the second version below. The adverbials, adjectives and prepositional phrases have been highlighted.

> *Florence Nightingale brought the people of the United Kingdom new ideas on medical practice. Without her experience in the Crimean war, the development of cleaner hospitals and improved training of nurses would not have benefited such a large number of people.*

2. What **kinds** of information and detail can adjectives, prepositional phrases and adverbials add to historical writing?

Improving an answer

3. Now look at the next section of this response below. How could you use prepositional phrases, adjectives and adverbs to make the response more precise and detailed? Use your own ideas or look at the comments for help.

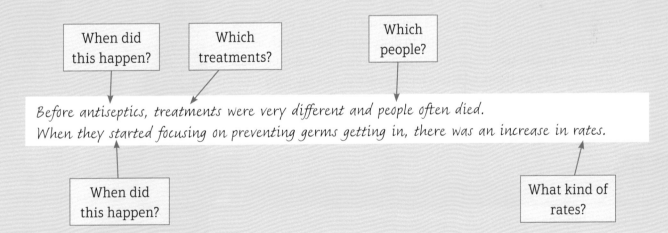

When did this happen? | Which treatments? | Which people?

Before antiseptics, treatments were very different and people often died.
When they started focusing on preventing germs getting in, there was an increase in rates.

When did this happen? | What kind of rates?

04 | c1900–present: Medicine in modern Britain

By 1900, all the pieces were in place to build a better approach to assessing and managing human health. People now understood that illness and disease could be caused by microbes, and scientists had begun to experiment with ways of treating and preventing diseases using this new knowledge.

Scientists began to investigate causes of disease that were not related to microbes. Genetics and lifestyle factors were investigated as other potential factors.

Chemical treatments were developed to target specific diseases, while antibiotics were discovered that could treat a whole range of illnesses that previously might have been fatal. Advances in surgical techniques made available life-saving treatments such as transplants.

The British government also developed a new attitude towards its role in the nation's health. Free medical care was provided for all through the National Health Service.

Unfortunately, understanding more about the causes of disease and illness has made us realise how much there is still to discover. Diseases such as cancer continue to puzzle scientists, who struggle to understand their cause or develop treatments for them. Lifestyle factors such as obesity have created new challenges for medicine to tackle. If the scientists of the 19th century had foreseen our progress, they would be amazed – however, the fight with disease is not yet over.

Learning outcomes

By the end of this chapter, you will:

- assess the changes in understanding the causes of illness and disease since 1900, including the impact of improved technology on diagnosis
- understand the changes in the treatment of disease
- assess the changes in medical treatment brought about by the introduction of the NHS and improvements in science and technology
- consider new approaches to the prevention of disease.
- understand how penicillin was discovered and developed.

4.1 Ideas about the cause of disease and illness

- Understand how advanced understanding of genetics and lifestyle choices affect health.
- Understand how improvements in technology have helped to improve diagnosis.

By 1900, Germ Theory had been around for nearly 40 years, and microbes had been clearly linked to outbreaks of disease. People finally understood what caused common diseases, such as cholera and diphtheria.

Because of this, throughout the 20th century, doctors no longer referred to miasmata, the Four Humours or the supernatural when diagnosing illness. This is the first period in which doctors were working solely with solid scientific discoveries. For the first time, they had more than just ideas about what caused diseases and illnesses – they had solid, evidence-based, knowledge.

At the start of the 20th century, diagnosis was something that happened between a doctor and a patient. The doctor would observe the patient and consider the symptoms. He would consult medical textbooks and diagnose the disease based on this knowledge.

During the 20th century, there was a move towards laboratory medicine, with more examination of **samples**. These samples might include skin or blood, or more detailed samples of flesh gathered from the patient in a procedure called a **biopsy**. The samples would be examined by medical scientists in a laboratory, using microscopes and other technology. In addition, the patient might be x-rayed to allow doctors to see what was going on inside the body, and the pictures produced would be examined by doctors looking for the cause of the disease or illness. All of this additional information meant that diagnosis was, and is, now more accurate. The exact microbe causing a disease can be identified and targeted.

Therefore, the biggest change in diagnosis in the 20th century was that, instead of being based on symptoms, and the experience and knowledge of the doctor, it was now based on medical testing.

Advances in understanding: the influence of genetic and lifestyle factors on health

The science of genetics

In 1900, it was clear to scientists that microbes did not cause all illnesses and diseases. For example, some babies were born with conditions that appeared to have developed in the womb.

This fact continued to stump doctors for the first half of the 20th century. It was clear that there was still a piece of the puzzle missing, related to the way that children inherited certain traits from their parents and how that related to hereditary diseases*.

Key term

Hereditary diseases*

Hereditary diseases are caused by genetic factors. This means that they can be passed on from parents to their children, or other descendants.

Early research into genetics

By 1900, a German scientist, Mendel, had theorised that genes come in pairs, and one is inherited from each parent. These were known as the **fundamental laws of inheritance**. Unfortunately, he did not have scientific proof that his laws were correct. Microscopes were not yet powerful enough to be able to identify gene pairs.

Timeline
Early work on genetics

1902 Archibald Garrod, an English doctor, theorises that hereditary diseases are caused by missing information in the body's chemical pathways.

1941 US scientists George Beadle and Edward Tatum prove Garrod's theory.

1951 At King's College in London, Rosalind Franklin and Maurice Wilkins create images of DNA using x-rays (see Source A).

Source A

Rosalind Franklin took this x-ray photograph of DNA in 1951 whilst working alongside Maurice Wilkins.

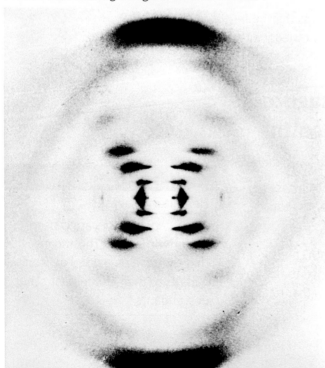

By 1951, scientists knew that characteristics were passed down from parents to children, as children often look like their parents. They theorised that a substance in human cells passed on this information from one person to the next. This substance also passed on a variety of hereditary diseases. However, it was not until 1953 that technology finally made it possible for scientists to find the missing piece of the puzzle: DNA*.

Key term

DNA*

Short for deoxyribonucleic acid, DNA carries genetic information from one living thing to another. DNA information determines characteristics like hair and eye colour.

Watson, Crick and the discovery of the human gene

James Watson was an American biologist. Francis Crick was an English physicist. In 1953, they were both working at Cambridge University, where they shared an office. Even though neither men were investigating DNA, they both had a strong interest in researching and finding out more about human biology.

Crick and Watson saw the x-rays provided by Franklin and Wilkins (see Source A). They built their model of DNA and shared it with Franklin, who made a correction based on her x-rays. Wilkins also shared clearer photographs that they had managed to take of the DNA. Due to this additional input, Crick and Watson were able to solve the puzzle of the structure of DNA. They discovered that it was shaped as a double helix, which could 'unzip' itself to make copies.

Watson and Crick published their paper in April 1953. Crick suggested that they had discovered the secret of life. Understanding the shape of DNA meant that they could now begin to look at its structure and identify the parts that caused hereditary diseases.

The mapping of the human genome*

Once the structure of DNA was understood, teams of scientists began to break it apart to understand how it worked. All the information that builds a person is stored in their DNA.

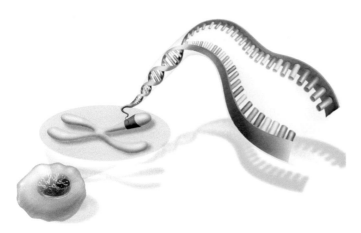

Figure 4.1 An image of the double helix formation of DNA. DNA is stored in every human cell.

Understanding that information – mapping the DNA's code – was vital to helping scientists understand the cause of genetic diseases, such as haemophilia*.

The Human Genome Project was launched in 1990. It was originally led by James Watson himself. For a decade, 18 teams of scientists all over the world worked together to decode and map the human genome. Even though hundreds of scientists were working towards this goal, they did not complete the first draft until 2000.

Once the human genome was mapped, it then became possible for scientists to use this blueprint of human DNA to look for mistakes or mismatches in the DNA of people suffering from hereditary diseases.

For example, scientists have now been able to identify a gene that is sometimes present in women who suffer from breast cancer. Although they cannot use this knowledge to **treat** breast cancer, women now have the opportunity to **prevent** this disease by identifying their risk of developing the disease and then having a mastectomy*. A famous example of this is the actress Angelina Jolie, who had herself tested for the gene because her mother had died of breast cancer.

Key terms

Genome*

The complete set of DNA containing all the information needed to build a particular organism. In humans, this is more than three billion DNA pairs. It is unique for every human being, except identical twins.

Haemophilia*

A genetic disease passed from parent to child that stops blood clotting. Sufferers from haemophilia must be careful, as an open wound will not heal correctly. Famously, many of Queen Victoria's ancestors suffered from haemophilia.

Mastectomy*

Surgery during which a person has one or both of their breasts removed.

Source B

In this 2013 news article, Angelina Jolie explains why she chose to have a mastectomy.

Angelina Jolie bravely reveals she has had a preventive double mastectomy after tests showed an 87% chance of contracting breast cancer.

The Hollywood actress is healthy and made the decision to undergo the procedure after discovering she carries the BRCA1 cancer gene.

Angelina said: "My doctors estimated that I had an 87% risk of breast cancer and a 50% risk of ovarian cancer. I made a decision to have a preventive double mastectomy."

The surgery was successful and doctors believe Angelina's chances of developing breast cancer have reduced to less than 5%.

Factors helping the development of genetics

Technology

Discovering the shape of DNA, understanding how it works and then mapping the individual genes has been made possible through improvements in technology. Advances in microscopes and the ability to produce higher-powered images enabled scientists to identify the DNA and then start to examine how it is formed.

The electron microscope was first developed in 1931 by a German physicist, Ernst Ruska, and electrical engineer, Max Knoll. Within two years, they had built a model that was able to magnify more than any of the optical microscopes that scientists had been using up to that point.

Electron microscopes work by using a beam of electrons to illuminate the sample being examined, instead of regular light. This allows for a much more powerful magnification. An optical microscope that uses visible light can clearly magnify a sample up to 2,000 times; an electron microscope can produce a clear image up to 10,000,000 times magnified.

Science

Understanding DNA required a lot of collaboration on the part of the scientific community. The Human Genome Project was an example of a new kind of 'big science' – thousands of scientists from all over the world collaborating to solve the same puzzle. All the data produced from the study was made public, so that it could benefit as many people as possible.

The impact of the science of genetics

A better understanding of DNA and how each part of the genome affects the body has helped scientists to recognise genetic disorders, such as Huntingdon's and Down's Syndrome. These disorders are caused by missing information in the genome: if that information can be put back in by scientists, this could theoretically lead to a treatment in some cases.

However, this is **not a current treatment**. A good understanding of genetics has helped doctors to better understand what causes diseases and illnesses, but the science is not yet at the stage where treatments of this nature are widely available for many diseases.

Activities ?

1 Create a chain of paper people. Each person should be a different figure that was important in the discovery of DNA. How many people can you make in your chain?

2 Explain why the discovery of the shape of DNA was so important for scientists.

3 Which factor was more important in the development of our understanding of genetics: science or technology? Write a short paragraph explaining your opinion.

Lifestyle and health

During the 20th century, we have gained a better understanding of the impact of lifestyle choices on the body and how these are linked with diseases and illnesses.

Smoking

Smoking became more popular from the 1920s. It was associated with being young and free. By the 1950s, doctors had started to notice a worrying rise in the number of men suffering from lung cancer, and this was linked with smoking (see page 122).

Doctors now recognise that smoking is associated with an enormous variety of diseases, including high blood pressure, a wide variety of cancers (including lung, throat and mouth), heart disease, and even gum disease and tooth decay. Smoking is the biggest cause of preventable diseases in the world. It is even dangerous to people who inhale the smoke second-hand. Studies show that children exposed to second-hand smoke are more likely to develop asthma than those who do not.

Diet

Due to the Theory of the Four Humours, our medieval ancestors believed that what we ate had a huge impact on our health. Although nobody believes this theory anymore, we now recognise that what you eat (and how much of it) has a huge impact on your health – but in very different ways to what was suggested in the Middle Ages.

Most people are probably familiar with the usual advice about a healthy diet: plenty of fresh fruits and vegetables, and most other things in moderation. Two particularly important substances when it comes to health are **sugar** and **fat**. Too much sugar can cause the body to develop type 2 diabetes. This is an incurable condition where the body is not able to process sugar in the bloodstream. Too much fat can lead to heart disease.

Not getting the right amount of nutrients or not eating enough at all can also cause health problems.

The influence of other lifestyle factors

- **Drinking too much alcohol**, either through binge drinking or drinking a lot over a long period of time, can lead to liver diseases and kidney problems.
- People now recognise that sharing bodily fluids with other people, either through **intravenous drug taking** or **unprotected sex**, can lead to the spread of certain diseases.
- The fashion for **tanning**, either naturally or using sun beds, has led to a rise in the number of cases of skin cancer worldwide.

Activities ?

1. Create flashcards to show different lifestyle factors and the disease that they may cause. Write the factor on one side and the associated illnesses on the other.

2. Using your flashcards, write an advice leaflet to explain threats to health.

3. How is your leaflet different from a leaflet that might have been made for people in the 15th century?

Improvements in diagnosis: the impact of the availability of blood tests, scans and monitors

New methods of diagnosis

The development of machines and computers has enabled doctors to have a better understanding of a patient's symptoms than in any previous time. For example, x-rays and CT scans (see Figure 4.2) mean that doctors no longer have to use surgery to diagnose all diseases.

The impact of technology

The enormous leap forward in technology since 1900 has made diagnosing disease much more accurate. This has, in turn, had a huge impact on doctors' ability to treat patients.

New methods of diagnosing disease are being developed all the time.

Source C

This article was published on the *Medical News Today* website in November 2015. It describes the use of a special type of dressing to help diagnose infection in burn patients.

Infections are the primary cause of complications in burn injuries, especially in children. Even a relatively mild hot water scald can readily become infected. Many deaths from burn injuries are due to sepsis [blood poisoning].

... Researchers at the University of Bath, in conjunction with the Healing Foundation Children's Burns Research Centre and the University of Brighton, have created a ground breaking solution to diagnosing wound infection. The team has developed a prototype dressing that changes colour when a wound becomes infected. The wound dressing on an uninfected area displays a discrete circular design. Within four hours of an infection, the colour and pattern change.

Exam-style question, Section B

Explain **one** way in which understanding of the causes of disease and illness was different in c1750 from the present day. **4 marks**

Exam tip

It is helpful to have a 'go-to' connective word to use here, to make sure you clearly demonstrate the change. 'Whereas' and 'however' are both good choices.

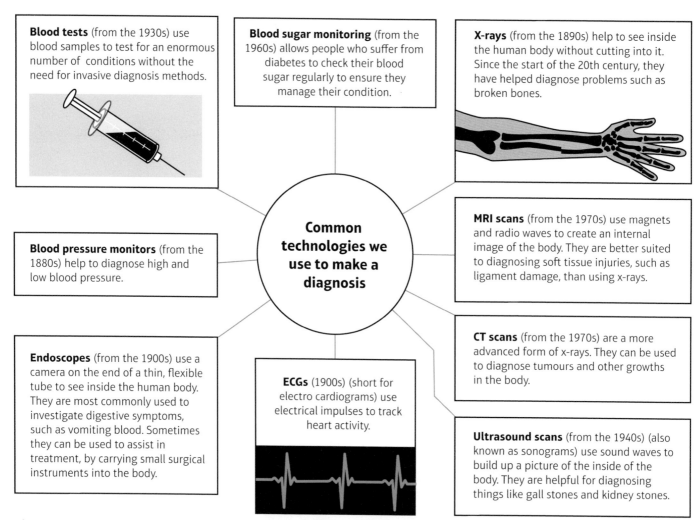

Blood tests (from the 1930s) use blood samples to test for an enormous number of conditions without the need for invasive diagnosis methods.

Blood sugar monitoring (from the 1960s) allows people who suffer from diabetes to check their blood sugar regularly to ensure they manage their condition.

X-rays (from the 1890s) help to see inside the human body without cutting into it. Since the start of the 20th century, they have helped diagnose problems such as broken bones.

Blood pressure monitors (from the 1880s) help to diagnose high and low blood pressure.

Common technologies we use to make a diagnosis

MRI scans (from the 1970s) use magnets and radio waves to create an internal image of the body. They are better suited to diagnosing soft tissue injuries, such as ligament damage, than using x-rays.

Endoscopes (from the 1900s) use a camera on the end of a thin, flexible tube to see inside the human body. They are most commonly used to investigate digestive symptoms, such as vomiting blood. Sometimes they can be used to assist in treatment, by carrying small surgical instruments into the body.

ECGs (1900s) (short for electro cardiograms) use electrical impulses to track heart activity.

CT scans (from the 1970s) are a more advanced form of x-rays. They can be used to diagnose tumours and other growths in the body.

Ultrasound scans (from the 1940s) (also known as sonograms) use sound waves to build up a picture of the inside of the body. They are helpful for diagnosing things like gall stones and kidney stones.

Figure 4.2 Common technologies developed in period 1900 – present to help diagnosis.

Summary

- After 1900, understanding about the causes of disease and illness progressed rapidly.
- By the end of the 20th century, doctors recognised that many factors caused disease.
- The structure of the gene was discovered by Watson and Crick in 1953 and the human genome was mapped by 2000.
- Lifestyle factors such as smoking, a poor diet and drinking alcohol can all contribute to illness and disease.
- New technology has enabled doctors to carry out more detailed diagnoses of their patients.

Checkpoint

Strengthen

S1 Explain how the mapping of the human genome helped doctors to better understand the causes of disease and illness.

S2 Describe three ways that technology has led to a better understanding of the causes of disease and illness.

Challenge

C1 How did changes in the way scientists work lead to an improved understanding of the causes of disease?

C2 Explain five examples of the impact of technology on diagnosing the causes of illness and disease.

If you are struggling, discuss the answers to these questions in groups. Your teacher can give you some hints.

4.2 Approaches to prevention and treatment

Medical treatments

The first chemical cures: magic bullets

The term 'magic bullet' was used to describe a chemical cure that would **attack the microbes in the body causing disease**, whilst at the same time **leaving the body unharmed**.

In the late 19th century, more microbes responsible for specific diseases were being discovered. This meant that scientists could begin to search for substances to attack and destroy these microbes.

Doctors now understood that the body produced **antibodies** to fight diseases that had previously infected it – this is how vaccines work. The hunt was on for artificial or chemical antibodies that would work in the same way, attacking the infection without harming the body.

The first big breakthrough was made in the treatment of syphilis. Syphilis continued to be a problem throughout the 19th and 20th centuries, and treatment of it had not really improved since mercury treatments of the 16th century. There had been some success with arsenic compounds*. However, it was very difficult to find a form of arsenic that attacked the disease and not the body, as arsenic is poisonous.

Key term

Compound*

A compound is a mixture of two or more different elements.

Extend your knowledge

Prontosil

Prontosil was used as a cure for puerperal fever at Queen Charlotte's maternity hospital in London. The death rate for puerperal fever dropped from 20% to 4.7%.

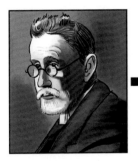 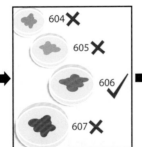 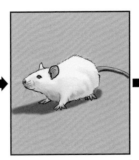 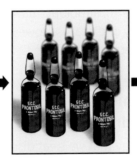 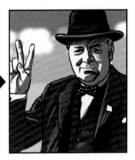

In the early 20th century, a scientist named Paul Ehrlich tested as many arsenic compounds as he could to find a cure for syphilis. By 1907, he had tested over 600 compounds, but had not found a cure.

In 1909, a Japanese scientist named Hata retested all of the compounds and found that compound number 606 cured syphilis. The drug, named Salvarsan 606, was the first 'magic bullet'.

In 1932, scientist Gerhard Domagk discovered that a bright red dye called Prontosil killed bacterial infections in mice. Domagk was forced to test Prontosil out on his own daughter, who had developed blood poisoning: it cured her.

Scientists at the Pasteur Institute in Paris discovered that Prontosil worked by preventing the bacteria from multiplying in the body. This made it possible for the body's own immune system to kill the bacteria. These drugs are called bacteriostatic antibiotics.

Scientists began to look for other drugs that worked in the same way. In 1938, British scientists developed M&B 693. This was another bacteriostatic antibiotic. It was successfully used to treat Winston Churchill for pneumonia during the Second World War.

Figure 4.3 The discovery of the first two magic bullets.

The development of antibiotics

The term **antibiotic** is used to describe any treatment that destroys or limits the growth of bacteria in the human body. The first true antibiotic was **penicillin**. Penicillin was different to Salvarsan 606 and Prontosil as it was created using microorganisms, not chemicals. Penicillin was isolated from a mould sample by Alexander Fleming in 1928 and developed into a usable treatment by Florey and Chain in 1940 (see pages 119–121).

Inspired by the discovery of penicillin, other scientists investigated moulds and fungi in the search for more antibiotics. Streptomycin was discovered by American scientist Selman Wakston in 1943. This antibiotic was so powerful that it was even effective against tuberculosis, which had previously been thought to be incurable. During the 1950s and 1960s, even more antibiotics were discovered.

Research into the development of new antibiotics has not stopped. In the 21st century, pharmaceutical companies continue to test substances to develop new antibiotics. This is because some bacteria have developed a resistance to the antibiotics we already have. If new treatments are not developed, scientists fear that the old antibiotics will become totally ineffective against diseases that we think we have beaten, such as septicaemia (blood poisoning).

Therefore, in the short term, antibiotics have been a miracle cure for a variety of diseases. However, their long-term impact has yet to be measured.

The impact of science and technology on advances in medicines

As with diagnosis, the way that we treat diseases now is almost unrecognisable from the way that people treated them before 1900. This is largely due to huge **advances in science and technology.**

Scientists have now developed medicines that pinpoint and treat specific diseases. Even if they are unable to cure some diseases, such as diabetes and lung cancer, treatments have been developed to help patients

Source A

This article, entitled *'Too much of a good thing'*, was published in *The Telegraph* in 2013, by Joe Shute.

Antibiotics are no longer effective. The drugs that have transformed life and longevity and saved countless millions since penicillin was discovered by Sir Alexander Fleming in 1928 now saturate [fill] every corner of our environment. We stuff them into ourselves and our animals; we spray them on crops, dump them in rivers, and even — as emerged at a meeting of science ministers from the G8 last year – paint them on the hulls of boats to keep off barnacles.

As a result, an invisible army of super-resistant bacteria has evolved, one that is increasingly claiming lives — currently more than 25,000 a year in Europe alone...

Many leading scientists and doctors and politicians are freely adopting the language of global catastrophe. Infections such as tuberculosis and septicaemia – the scourge of earlier centuries – are once again killing us at frightening rates. We have used, or are using, our so-called drugs of last resort.

manage their illness. Scientists are now able to identify the causes of disease in most cases, because they know what they are looking for – for example, a microbe, a tumour or an unusual gene. This is a huge change from the 19th century.

Improved scientific understanding has also led to better testing and trialling of new treatments before they are given to patients. In the past, drugs did not have to go through this process before being used to treat disease. This meant that mistakes were made. The most famous of these mistakes was the use of the drug thalidomide in the 1960s to treat pregnant women suffering from morning sickness. The drug caused birth defects.

Now, it takes several years for a new drug to be trialled thoroughly before being used. This slows down progress but ensures drugs are safe for everybody.

THINKING HISTORICALLY Change and continuity (4b&c)

The bird's eye view

Development	Example of immediate changes	Example of change in the medium term	Example of change in the long term
The development of antibiotics		Scientists developed a way of making antibiotics, which meant they could be modified to attack particular diseases.	Antibiotics are still used widely to treat diseases and infections. However, there are an increasing number of diseases that are resistant to them.

Imagine you are looking at the whole of history using a zoomed-out interactive map like Google Maps™. You have a general view of the sweep of developments and their consequences, but you cannot see much detail. If you zoom in to the time when antibiotics were first developed, you can see the event in detail but will know nothing of its consequences in the medium or long term.

Look at the table above and answer the following:

1   What were the immediate changes brought about by the development of antibiotics? Write down at least two changes that could complete that column in the table.

2   Look at the medium-term changes and the long-term changes. How are they similar? How are they different?

3   Work in groups of three. Each take the role of the teacher for one of the above (the immediate changes, the medium-term changes or the long-term changes). Give a short presentation to the other two students in your group, explaining the key changes over your timescale. They may comment and ask questions.

Answer the following individually:

4   How was your explanation of change different to the other explanations? Write a short paragraph using examples from what you and the rest of your group said.

5   What happens to the detail, particularly of the medium- and short-term changes, when you zoom out to look at the long-term changes?

6   What are the advantages and disadvantages of zooming in to look at a specific time in detail?

New technology has made it easier to create and provide drugs to treat diseases.

- **Mass production of pills** has made the distribution of drugs much easier.
- **The development of capsules**, which dissolve in the stomach to release the drug, means taking drugs to treat disease is easier.
- **Hypodermic needles** allow the precise dose to be introduced directly into the bloodstream.
- **Insulin pumps** for young people suffering from diabetes deliver insulin without the need for injections.

Activities ?

1   Draw a timeline to show when the different drugs described in this section were developed. Label each one with details, such as who was responsible for its development and which diseases the drug fights.

2   Describe how science and technology assisted in the development of new chemical treatments.

3   Individuals like Ehrlich and Domagk inspired British scientists to look for new treatments, while science and technology made them possible. Which factor do you think has been the most important in the development of treatments post-1900?

Medical care: impact of the NHS

Phase one: Improved access to care

The National Health Service (NHS) was launched in 1948 by the government. Its aim was to provide medical care for the entire population of Britain. It was paid for by National Insurance contributions, taken from wages in the same way as tax. It was the largest government intervention in medical care. The new NHS took over existing hospitals and medical services.

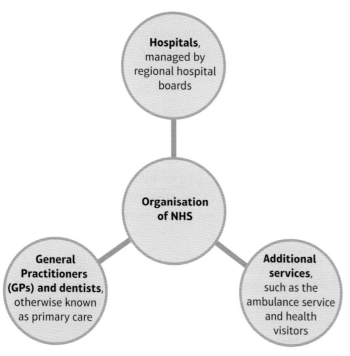

Figure 4.4 The three parts of the NHS in 1948.

The government aimed to provide the same level of service for everybody in the country, no matter how rich or poor they were.

For example, workers earning under a certain amount were already entitled to medical care through the 1911 National Insurance Act. However, this did not extend to women who were at home raising their families. After 1948, women were able to get treatment for painful conditions like varicose veins, which might previously have been left untreated. Similarly, children could be treated for minor problems before there was any lasting damage.

To begin with, hospitals were not much changed by the launch of the NHS. Post-war Britain did not have a lot of money to spend on medical care. The government was now responsible for 1,143 voluntary hospitals and 1,545 city hospitals, which was a huge undertaking. Many of the hospitals had been built in the 19th century and desperately needed updating. There were also more hospitals in London and the South East than there were across the rest of the country.

Similarly, many GP surgeries were in need of modernisation, as well as the standards of the GPs themselves. Studies in the 1950s suggested that up to a quarter of GPs were not satisfactory. With little time or opportunity to keep up-to-date with medical developments, many GPs were behind the times. The problem was made worse by the NHS, because more and more people began visiting GPs. Waiting times increased and appointment times decreased.

Therefore, **access had improved** because the NHS was available to all. However, **provision had not improved** in the short term. During the 1960s, however, the government implemented changes to improve the NHS. Plans were made to ensure that hospitals were evenly spread across the whole country. In 1966, a GP's charter was introduced, which encouraged GPs to work in group practices and gave them incentives to keep up with medical developments. The government had to manage the NHS rather than just fund it. This led to improvements in the standard of care.

Phase two: High-tech medical and surgical treatments in hospitals

Hospital treatments have changed a lot since 1900. Treatments that we consider routine today, like hip replacements and blood transfusions, did not exist before 1900. Patients benefit from high-tech treatments that would have been unimaginable in previous centuries. Once the three major problems of surgery – **pain, infection and blood loss** – had been solved, doctors were able to carry out more daring and intrusive surgeries than ever before. The development of new machinery to treat the body and even replace parts of it that had stopped working also improved treatment in hospitals.

There are hundreds of examples of new high-tech medical and surgical treatments being carried out. The table opposite shows a few of the most famous examples.

	New technology	Treatment made possible
Medical treatments	Advanced x-rays	Doctors can now also use x-rays to target and shrink tumours growing inside the body, using a treatment known as **radiotherapy**. Combined with chemotherapy, this is an effective treatment for many types of cancer.
	Smaller, cheaper machines	Processes like **dialysis**, where the blood of patients with kidney failure is 'washed' by a machine, and **heart bypasses**, where a machine performs the functions of the heart, have become more widely available as machines have become smaller and more portable.
	Robotics	Better **prosthetic limbs** are now produced. This is partly in response to the number of soldiers surviving bomb attacks in recent wars in Iraq and Afghanistan.
Surgical treatments	Microsurgery	The first successful kidney transplant was performed between identical twins in the USA in 1956. This paved the way for transplants of other organs, including lungs (from 1963), and livers and hearts (from 1967). These were made possible by improved surgical techniques, including the use of microsurgery to reattach tiny nerve endings and blood vessels.
	Laparoscopic (keyhole) surgery	Using tiny cameras and narrow surgical instruments, surgeons can now operate inside the body through tiny incisions some distance away from the area to be operated on. This allows for quicker healing and less trauma to the body.
	Robotic surgery	Surgeons can now use computers to control instruments inside the body, allowing for more precise surgery with smaller cuts. Operations can be performed on a tiny scale where precision is of vital importance – for example, in brain surgery.

Interpretation 1

In this interpretation, taken from *Health and Medicine in Britain since 1860* by Anne Hardy (2001), the short-term impact of the NHS is called into question.

The implementation of the NHS by no means resolved the problem of delivering adequate health care to Britain's people, although it did offer a considerable improvement over the combination of private and insurance medicine that had preceded it. The medical services offered under the 1948 Act were pre-eminently providers of treatment for existing illness rather than agents for preventing its development.

Extend your knowledge

3D printers
At the cutting edge of medical research, scientists are attempting to develop a way of creating new organs using 3D printers. However, this is still decades away from being a usable treatment.

Interpretation 2

Former Labour Prime Minister Tony Blair wrote this as part of a foreword to a document about the modernisation of the NHS. It was published in 1997.

Creating the NHS was the greatest act of modernisation ever achieved by a Labour Government. It banished the fear of becoming ill that had for years blighted the lives of millions of people.

The extent of change in care and treatment

Treatment

Looking back to the 17th century, when Thomas Sydenham imagined a world in which each disease would have its own treatment, the change in the way diseases have been treated is immense.

In the 20th century, medical science made a huge leap forward towards Sydenham's dream. In 1900, 25% of deaths were caused by infectious diseases. By 1990, that number had fallen to less than 1%.

In c1900, most people were still taking herbal remedies or patent medicines, such as Beechams, bought from the chemist to treat their illnesses. Now, thanks to advances in science after 1900, there are a wide variety of specific, effective medicines matched with the diseases that they treat.

However, scientists continue to face problems when developing treatments.

- It is very difficult to develop a vaccine against some viruses. A different flu vaccine is available every year, as scientists develop it in response to the most common strain of the flu virus at that time.

- New diseases keep appearing, which do not respond to any chemical treatments that we currently know about. Scientists have to go back to the lab and continue testing compounds in the hope that they might find one that is effective.

- Lifestyle factors have caused an increase in illnesses such as heart disease and cancer, for which there are no certain cures.

- Microbes are living organisms and they have evolved to beat some of the cures doctors have been using. This has led to drug-resistant bacteria, such as MRSA*. Tuberculosis cases are once again on the rise in the UK.

We may not be facing all the same problems as our ancestors when researching treatments for illness and disease, but we face many new ones. Therefore, alternative remedies, such as herbal medicines, acupuncture and homeopathy, are still popular treatments for disease.

Improved access to care

In c1900, most sick people were still cared for in the home by women. Doctors had to be paid and so were only used for serious illnesses.

The situation improved slowly during the first half of the 20th century. In 1919, the government set up the Ministry of Health to help determine the level of health care across the country.

There was rapid improvement in the availability of care outside the home from 1948 onwards. The NHS made medical services free at point of service. This gave everybody access to medical care and treatment.

However, the introduction of the NHS made it clear, once and for all, that hospitals were just for treating the sick. In earlier periods, hospitals had been places for the elderly to rest. This change left a gap in services. Up until the end of the Second World War, elderly people with no family had often lived out the last days of their life in hospitals. This was no longer possible.

Exam-style question, Section B

'Treatment of diseases and care of the sick completely changed after c1800'.

How far do you agree with this statement?

You may use the following information in your answer:

- magic bullets
- the NHS.

You **must** also use information of your own. **16 marks**

Exam tip

Focus on the word 'completely' in this question. Nobody would argue that treatment and care has stayed the same since c1800, so in your answer you should focus on whether it is entirely different or whether there are some things that are the same as previous centuries.

Key term

MRSA*

A strain of drug-resistant bacteria that is particularly hardy and resistant to antibiotics.

Activity

Draw a table to show the change and change continuity in care and treatment from earlier periods to the end of the 19th century.

Preventing disease

By c1900, many different approaches to preventing disease had been put in place. The government now took responsibility for providing clean water and removing waste. The public understood the importance of these factors, due to the development of Germ Theory. As more people were given the vote, the government paid more attention to what its citizens wanted.

The government has taken significant action to improve the public's health since the beginning of the 20th century. The *laissez-faire* attitude was now behind them. There are two reasons for this.

1 Increased understanding of cause

Now that we understand what causes disease, the government recognises that its intervention can have an impact. Without this understanding, the British government would not have acted in the same way, because they did not know that their intervention could change things.

2 Increased understanding of methods of prevention

Once the causes of disease and health problems was understood, methods of prevention could be tested and introduced. These have included:

- **Compulsory vaccinations:** inspired by the positive impact of the smallpox vaccination, other campaigns were launched in the 20th century.

- **Passing laws to provide a healthy environment:** these include the Clean Air Acts (see page 114) and adding the chemical fluoride to the water supply to help prevent tooth decay.

- **Communicating health risks:** lifestyle campaigns help people to identify and tackle health risks. During times of global epidemics, such as during the 2014–15 outbreak of ebola in West Africa, the government tracked travellers from affected regions and put quarantine measures in place to stop the spread of disease. Communicating risks to the population has become key in preventing disease.

Charities also contribute to healthy lifestyle campaigns. For example, the British Heart Foundation creates adverts encouraging people to protect their heart by giving up smoking, eating less fat and exercising.

New approaches to prevention: mass vaccinations

Timeline

Government introduction of vaccinations

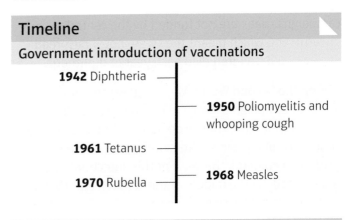

1942 Diphtheria

1950 Poliomyelitis and whooping cough

1961 Tetanus

1968 Measles

1970 Rubella

Source B

This poster advertising diphtheria immunisation was published in 1943, one year after the national campaign was launched.

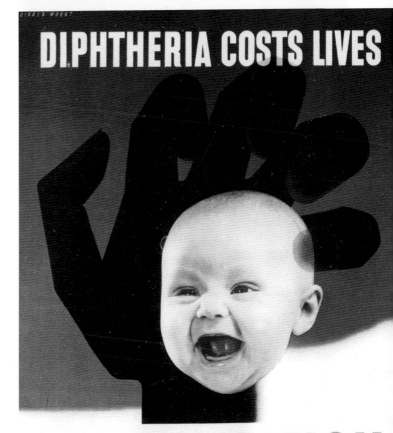

DIPHTHERIA COSTS LIVES

IMMUNISATION COSTS NOTHING

The national vaccination campaign against diphtheria was launched in 1942 – the first of its kind. Before this, local governments were responsible for vaccination campaigns that were not funded by the central government, which meant they were not widespread. Around 3,000 children died each year of diphtheria.

During the Second World War, the government put a national campaign in place to immunise all children against diphtheria. There were fears that the cramped conditions of air-raid shelters during the war might lead to an epidemic. Because of this, infection rates plummeted. By the middle of the century, diphtheria was seen as a disease of the past.

Another significant vaccination campaign was against poliomyelitis (polio). Polio is a very contagious disease that causes paralysis. In the early 1950s, there were as many as 8,000 cases reported every year in Britain. The vaccination was developed in the USA by Jonas Salk and was introduced to the UK in 1956, followed by a more effective vaccination in 1962. As with diphtheria, the number of infections dropped very rapidly. The last case of a person contracting polio in the UK was in 1984.

Some vaccines are aimed at protecting future generations. Rubella, or German measles, is not a life-threatening disease for most people – however, it can be very dangerous if a pregnant woman catches it because it will affect the unborn child.

Other vaccines target diseases that can lead to other diseases. The HPV vaccine, for example, protects women against infection from a sexually transmitted disease that has been linked to cervical cancer.

There continues to be controversy surrounding vaccinations. Many people resent government intervention and choose not to vaccinate their children. A lack of trust in the medical profession has led to fears that vaccines are unsafe. While vaccination is the best way to prevent the spread of dangerous epidemic diseases, there is still freedom of choice to reject this method.

New approaches to prevention: government legislation

The government has passed laws to provide a healthy environment for the population. Examples of these were the Clean Air Acts of 1956 and 1968. They were triggered by bad episodes of smog in London in 1952.

Smog is very heavy fog caused by air pollution. In an era a time when everybody burned coal to heat their homes, there was a great deal of smoke and soot in the air, particularly in London, where a lot of people lived. Sometimes there was so much pollution that smog would cover the city for days at a time.

Smog is no longer a significant problem in the UK. However, the government continues to pass laws to protect the population from air pollution. An example of this is by limiting car emissions.

Source C

Lavinia Hand was born in London in 1924. During the Great Smog she lived with her husband, George, and their two-year-old son Peter. Here she recollects the conditions.

```
It was really a very terrible fog. Everybody
had coal or wood fires at that time so there
was a lot of soot in the air, but it was
traffic pollution as well. The air was so
dangerous that thousands of people died.
We lived in Wood Green and George worked in
Finchley. He wore a mask but the smog made our
eyes sting as well and the mask didn't help
with that. I wouldn't take Peter out in it.
```

The government have also passed legislation making it illegal to smoke in all enclosed workplaces. It came into force on 1 July 2007 as part of the Health Act of 2006.

Source D

A picture of a London policeman wearing a facemask in the last London smog, in 1962. Pharmacists sold masks like this to help people avoid the negative effects of breathing in the pollution.

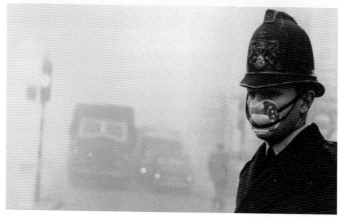

New approaches to prevention: government lifestyle campaigns

As well as providing direct intervention to prevent disease, the government also aims to help people prevent disease themselves, by promoting healthier lifestyles. Some examples of their work include:

- advertising campaigns warning against dangers to health, such as smoking, binge drinking, recreational drug use and unprotected sex
- events such as Stoptober, which encourage people to stop smoking for a month
- initiatives encouraging people to eat more healthily and get more exercise, such as the Change4Life campaign (see Source E).

Source E

A poster published by Change4Life in 2015. Change4Life is a Public Health England campaign designed to help families eat well and move more.

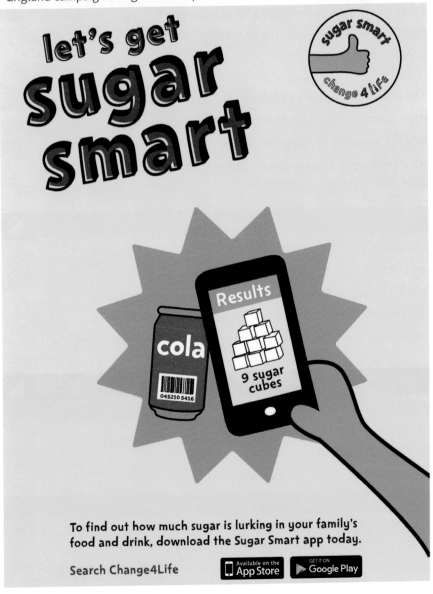

Exam-style question, Section B

Explain why there was rapid progress in disease prevention after c1900.

You may use the following in your answer:

- government intervention
- vaccinations.

You **must** also use information of your own. **12 marks**

Exam tip

Remember that all of that knowledge needs to **support** your arguments – avoid simply describing disease prevention.

> ### THINKING HISTORICALLY — Cause and Consequence (2a)
>
> **The web of multiple causes**
>
> **Why were doctors able to treat more diseases in the 20th century?**
>
> Study these causes that would help historians to explain why doctors were able to treat diseases successfully in the 20th century.
>
> | | | |
> |---|---|---|
> | Fleming, Florey and Chain had developed penicillin, which led to the discovery of other antibiotics. | Technology such as x-rays made it easier for doctors to identify the specific causes of disease. | Everybody now understood and accepted that many diseases were caused by microbes. |
> | Scientists had isolated the microbes that caused different diseases. | Chemical cures, such as chemical 'magic bullets', had been developed. | The NHS provided medical care that was free at point of service. |
>
> Work in pairs. Take an A3 sheet of paper. You will need to use all of this.
>
> 1   Write two of the causes on the paper with some space between them.
> 2   Think of anything that connects the causes, draw a line between them and describe the connection by writing along the line.
> 3   Add all the other causes in turn and make as many links as you can with other causes.
> 4   Now add the outcome to the diagram: 'People believed in Germ Theory'. Think carefully about where to place this and how it should be linked into the diagram of causes.
>
> Answer the following:
>
> 5   Explain why it would be difficult to put the above causes on a timeline.
> 6   Which of the causes have an effect on other causes? Which are linked directly to the outcome?
> 7   Can your diagram help you to work out which causes were more important?
> 8   Write a paragraph explaining why doctors were able to treat diseases successfully in the 20th century. Make sure you mention all the causes in the table. Use the links you have identified between the causes to help you.

Summary

- Penicillin was discovered and then developed into a usable treatment for a wide variety of diseases.
- New technology helped to improve the way that medicines were given to patients.
- The government established the NHS in 1948. This made free medical care available to everybody.
- High-tech treatments, such as organ transplants and radiotherapy, helped doctors tackle diseases.
- Government sponsored campaigns encouraged people to lead healthier lives in order to prevent disease.

Checkpoint

Strengthen

S1 Choose three pieces of new technology and explain how they have helped to treat disease.

S2 What impact did the NHS have on the health of the nation?

S3 List five methods of preventing disease that have appeared since c1900.

Challenge

C1 Which factor do you think has had the biggest impact on treatment and prevention since 1900: government or science and technology? Select at least three examples from the text to support your answer.

Before writing your answer to question C1, you might find it useful to create a mind map listing your examples.

4.3 Fleming, Florey and Chain's development of penicillin

Learning outcomes

- Understand how Fleming, Florey and Chain discovered and developed penicillin.
- Understand how penicillin is used to treat diseases.

Following the development of the first 'magic bullet' in 1909, the search for effective treatments continued throughout the 20th century. The development of penicillin into a usable drug revolutionised the way that infections were combated and has saved countless lives.

Timeline

The development of penicillin

1928 Fleming identifies penicillin in his lab.

1929 Fleming publishes his findings.

1939 Florey and Chain revive Fleming's research.

1940 Florey and Chain successfully treat mice with penicillin.

1941 Florey and Chain trial penicillin on a human, with some success.

1942 US pharmaceutical companies begin mass producing penicillin.

1945 Dorothy Crowfoot Hodgkin, a scientist at Oxford University, identifies the chemical structure of penicillin.

1957 Chemist John C. Sheehan creates a chemical copy of penicillin. This allows for the drug to be changed in order to target different diseases.

Alexander Fleming and the discovery of penicillin

Alexander Fleming was a British doctor working at St Mary's Hospital in London. He had a particular interest in bacteriology and had been one of the first doctors to use the first 'magic bullet' to treat syphilis. During the First World War, Fleming had worked in battlefield hospitals trying to improve treatments for wounded soldiers. He was dismayed at the number of men who died from simple infections.

During the 1920s, Fleming researched substances that might be effective in combating these simple infections. In 1928, he noticed something unusual about his dirty petri dishes: one of them had developed some mould. The mould appeared to have killed off the harmful staphylococcus bacteria that had been growing in the dish.

Fleming tested the mould and identified it as penicillin. He was not the first person to notice what it could do: in the Middle Ages, people were aware that mouldy bread had healing properties, and Joseph Lister used it to treat a patient in 1871. However, Fleming published his findings at a time when scientists were actively looking for chemical treatments for disease, and so more notice was taken of it.

Unfortunately, Fleming did not believe that penicillin could work to kill bacteria in living people. His first experiments with the mould showed that it became ineffective when mixed with blood in test tubes in the laboratory, so he did not pursue funding to perform further tests on the mould.

Source A

A photograph of a plaque on the wall of St Mary's Hospital in Paddington, London, commemorating Fleming's achievement.

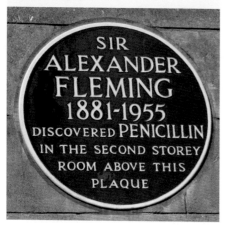

Source B

A photograph of Alexander Fleming studying mould cultures in his laboratory at the Wright Fleming Institute in London.

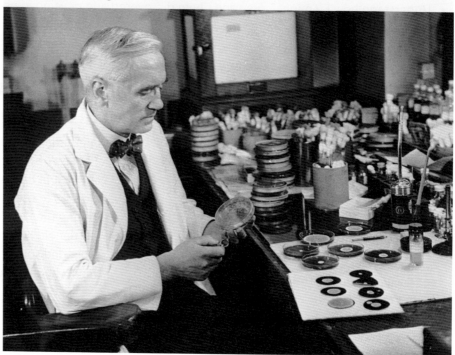

Source C

In 1945, Alexander Fleming was awarded the Nobel Prize in Medicine for his discovery of penicillin. He shared this with Howard Florey and Ernst Chain. In this extract from his acceptance speech, Alexander Fleming describes the process of discovering the antibiotic.

In 1928 an accidental contamination of a culture plate by a mould set me off on another track. I was working on a subject having no relation to moulds or antiseptics and if I had been a member of a team engaged on this subject it is likely that I would have had to neglect the accidental happening and work for the team with the result that penicillin would not then have been described and I would not be here today as a Nobel Laureate...

... I isolated the contaminating mould. It made an antibacterial substance which I christened penicillin. I studied it as far as I could as a bacteriologist. I had a clue that here was something good but I could not possibly know how good it was and I had not the team, especially the chemical team, necessary to concentrate and stabilise the penicillin.

Florey and Chain and the development of penicillin

Howard Florey was an Australian pathologist working at Oxford medical school. His colleague, Ernst Chain, had escaped Nazi Germany, where he had been a biochemist.

Florey and Chain were conducting research in the field of antibiotics. As part of this, they were looking for neglected research that might be worth investigating. They came across Fleming's findings and decided that the mould should be tested further. Chain grew the mould in his laboratory and used extracts of it in tests for treatment.

In 1940, Florey and Chain tested their extracted penicillin on infected mice. The results were promising: it looked as though the penicillin was killing the infection. Unfortunately, it was very difficult to produce penicillin in large quantities. The active ingredient in the liquid produced by the mould only represented one part per two million – that meant growing a great deal of mould before it was possible to get started on a human trial.

The scientists set about growing as much penicillin as possible. They used whatever they could to grow the mould: milk churns, bed pans and even a bath tub. By 1941, Florey and Chain had a human patient on whom to try the drug: a local policeman who had developed an infection. He had been scratched by a rose bush and had developed septicaemia – fatal blood poisoning.

Florey and Chain only had a very small amount of penicillin, but they gave it to the policeman anyway. He showed signs of recovery almost straight away. However, there had not been enough penicillin to cure him completely and there was no more available. Florey and Chain collected the patient's urine and extracted leftover penicillin from it. This was then given to the patient and, again, he showed signs of getting better. Unfortunately, this could only be done so many times and the patient eventually died.

Nevertheless, penicillin had proved to be effective in fighting infection in the human body.

Interpretation 1

There is some controversy over who should get the credit for the development of penicillin. In this study of the role of science in science education, published in 1996, Patricia Harding sets out an alternative point of view.

Fleming did not develop penicillin. He found it in 1928, extracted it from a culture of [the mould] *Penicillium*, and worked on it for a short time. By 1931 he had abandoned it as an antiseptic for medical use and used it only as an ingredient in culture medium to selectively grow certain organisms. Penicillin was developed therapeutically in 1940 by a group of scientists at Oxford under the leadership of Howard Florey. However, when penicillin made such an impact on the world, Fleming managed to get the credit, and the group at Oxford were ignored by the public. Early accounts propagated [spread] the "myth" of the development of penicillin, but several scientists who knew what had happened later told the real story.

THINKING HISTORICALLY — Change and continuity (4a)

Significance

Look at Source C on page 118 and Interpretation 1 above.

1 In what ways does Fleming think he was significant in the discovery of penicillin?

2 How significant does Fleming feel he was in the discovery of penicillin?

3 Compare this to historian Patricia Harding. What significance does Harding credit to Fleming?

4 Why do you think these views might differ so greatly?

Activity ?

Discuss Interpretation 1 with a partner. Why does Patricia Harding feel that Fleming should not get the credit for penicillin?

Mass production of penicillin

Florey and Chain proved that penicillin was effective in treating infections, but they were still struggling to mass produce it. They needed a large-scale factory where the penicillin could be grown and extracted on an industrial scale.

Florey first approached British pharmaceutical companies for assistance. Unfortunately, this was during the Second World War and the companies were busy producing materials for the war effort.

However, the USA had not yet joined the war. In July 1941, Florey visited the USA and convinced pharmaceutical companies to begin penicillin production. The companies started growing the penicillin in beer vats. It was a very slow process – after a year, the US companies only had enough penicillin to treat ten people.

However, once this had begun, the impact of penicillin could be shown. The US government, observing the benefits of the drug, funded 21 pharmaceutical companies to begin mass producing it. British pharmaceutical companies became involved in 1943, when they too started to mass produce the drug. By D-Day, in June 1944, there was enough penicillin available to treat all Allied casualties.

Factors enabling the development of penicillin

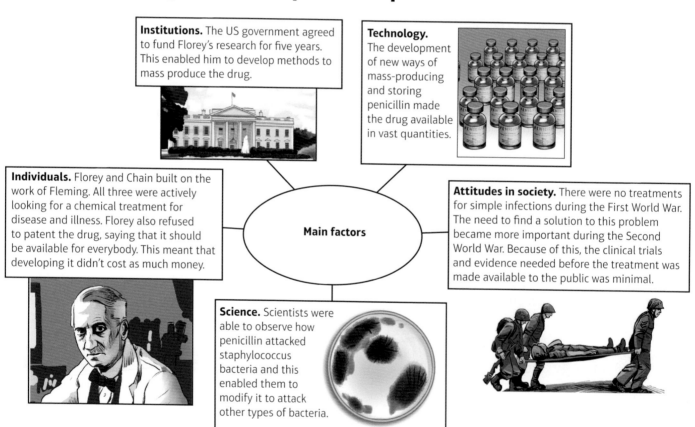

Institutions. The US government agreed to fund Florey's research for five years. This enabled him to develop methods to mass produce the drug.

Technology. The development of new ways of mass-producing and storing penicillin made the drug available in vast quantities.

Individuals. Florey and Chain built on the work of Fleming. All three were actively looking for a chemical treatment for disease and illness. Florey also refused to patent the drug, saying that it should be available for everybody. This meant that developing it didn't cost as much money.

Main factors

Attitudes in society. There were no treatments for simple infections during the First World War. The need to find a solution to this problem became more important during the Second World War. Because of this, the clinical trials and evidence needed before the treatment was made available to the public was minimal.

Science. Scientists were able to observe how penicillin attacked staphylococcus bacteria and this enabled them to modify it to attack other types of bacteria.

Figure 4.5 The main factors that enabled the development of penicillin.

Use of penicillin

Penicillin is effective in treating diseases caused by a certain family of bacteria.

Penicillin is also used to **prevent** infection, particularly with patients who have had teeth extracted.

The development of penicillin also encouraged scientists to look for other moulds that could be used to fight bacterial infections – such as streptomycin, which was the first drug found to be effective against tuberculosis. Once Dorothy Hodgkin had mapped the chemical structure of penicillin (see the timeline, on page 117), scientists were able to begin working on

synthetic versions of it that were slightly modified to treat specific diseases.

Now that doctors could offer treatments that worked against a wide range of illnesses, confidence in medical treatments began to rise. Patients were more willing to seek out medical treatments from doctors.

Unfortunately, as explained on page 112, some bacteria are now resistant to penicillin. Bacteria can mutate to resist attack from penicillin mould. The first penicillin-resistant strain of bacteria appeared in 1942. Pharmaceutical companies continue to work hard to develop new forms of penicillin and other antibiotics that will kill off the bacteria.

Summary

- Alexander Fleming discovered penicillin by accident in 1928. His research went unnoticed until 1938, when it was developed by Howard Florey and Ernst Chain.
- Florey and Chain were able to create a usable drug from the mould, which they tested on mice and then a human being. However, it was very difficult to mass produce.
- When the Second World War broke out, Florey was able to secure funding from the US government to mass produce the drug.
- Penicillin is effective against a wide range of illnesses.

Checkpoint

Strengthen

S1 Describe the process by which Fleming discovered penicillin.

S2 How did Florey and Chain test penicillin when they isolated it?

S3 How did attitudes in society lead to the development of penicillin?

S4 How was penicillin developed after the Second World War?

Challenge

C1 How was the discovery of penicillin linked to:

- government intervention
- science and technology?

C2 With a partner, discuss the roles played by Fleming, Florey and Chain in the discovery and development of penicillin. Was it the right decision to award them the Nobel Prize jointly?

Discuss the answer to C1 in groups if you are struggling. Your teacher can give you some hints.

4.4 The fight against lung cancer in the 21st century

Learning outcomes

- Understand why lung cancer has become more widespread since the 19th century.
- Understand how science and technology has helped in diagnosing and treating lung cancer.
- Understand how the government has tried to prevent lung cancer.

Lung cancer is the second most common cancer in the UK. It mainly affects people over the age of 40, with diagnoses being highest among people aged 70–74.

Most lung cancers are caused by external factors. Around 85% of cases are people who smoke, or have smoked. Other chemicals in the air, such as radon gas, are also sometimes to blame. However, a small number of people develop lung cancer for no apparent reason.

There were very few cases of lung cancer discovered in the 19th century. Records kept at the University of Dresden in Germany, for example, show that only 1% of all cancers they found at autopsy were caused by lung tumours. However, by 1918, that had increased to 10%, and by 1927 it was more than 14%.

In 1950, the British Medical Research Council published a study that showed conclusively that the rise in lung cancer was linked to cigarette smoking. Aggressive advertising by the tobacco companies since the First World War had led to a huge rise in the number of smokers. In spite of the results of the study, deaths among men from lung cancer continued to rise. They peaked in 1973 when nearly 26,000 deaths occurred due to lung cancer. The death rate among women also continued to rise until the 1990s.

The use of science and technology in diagnosis

One of the reasons why lung cancer is so hard to treat is that usually, by the time the cancer is detected, it is already very advanced. Patients often mistake their symptoms for other diseases. There is no national screening programme for lung cancer, so people are not routinely tested to see if they have it. This is because the tests are not accurate enough to outweigh the negative effects of the screening (for example, exposure to radiation during an x-ray scan).

Diagnosis is also difficult, although technology has led to improvements in this area.

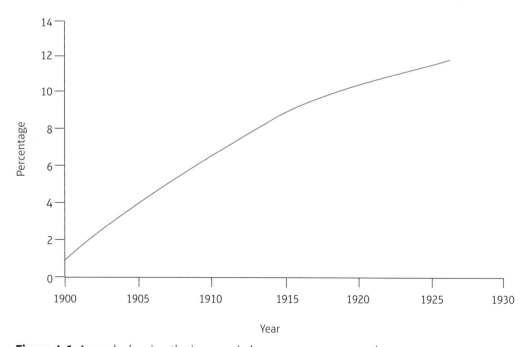

Figure 4.6 A graph showing the increase in lung cancer cases over time.

Diagnosing lung cancer

Before more advanced technology had been discovered, lung cancer was diagnosed using an x-ray machine. A doctor would examine the x-ray to look for a tumour.

This way of diagnosing was not ideal. Often other things, like lung abscesses, might be mistaken for cancer – or, worse, cancer could be mistaken for something less threatening. X-rays were not detailed enough to accurately diagnose cancer.

Figure 4.7 shows how lung cancer is diagnosed today.

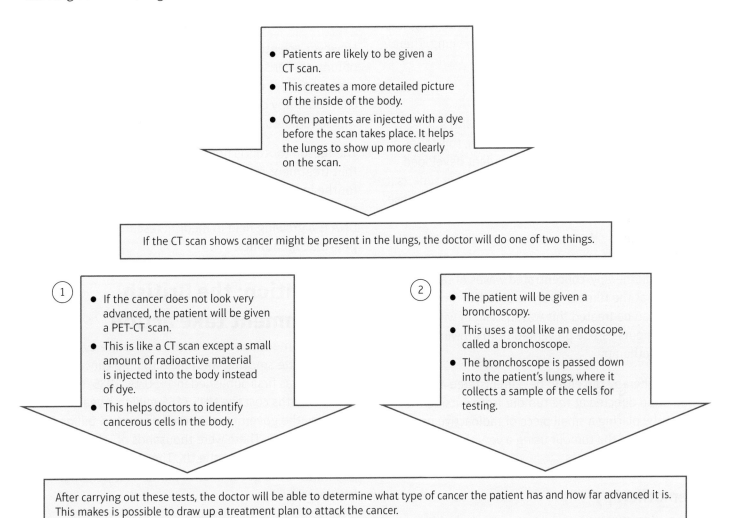

- Patients are likely to be given a CT scan.
- This creates a more detailed picture of the inside of the body.
- Often patients are injected with a dye before the scan takes place. It helps the lungs to show up more clearly on the scan.

If the CT scan shows cancer might be present in the lungs, the doctor will do one of two things.

1
- If the cancer does not look very advanced, the patient will be given a PET-CT scan.
- This is like a CT scan except a small amount of radioactive material is injected into the body instead of dye.
- This helps doctors to identify cancerous cells in the body.

2
- The patient will be given a bronchoscopy.
- This uses a tool like an endoscope, called a bronchoscope.
- The bronchoscope is passed down into the patient's lungs, where it collects a sample of the cells for testing.

After carrying out these tests, the doctor will be able to determine what type of cancer the patient has and how far advanced it is. This makes is possible to draw up a treatment plan to attack the cancer.

Figure 4.7 The stages of diagnosing lung cancer.

Activities ?

1 Explain the most common causes of lung cancer.

2 Explain why lung cancer is difficult to treat.

3 How has science and technology helped in the diagnosis of lung cancer?

The use of science and technology in lung cancer treatment

If lung cancer is diagnosed early, doctors can perform an operation to remove the tumour and the infected portion of the lung. This can range from the removal of just a small piece, to the removal of the entire lung. It is possible to breathe normally with only one lung. There are also other treatments to consider.

Transplants

It is possible to replace cancerous lungs with a transplant from a healthy donor. However, this raises a number of ethical problems if the patient developed lung cancer after smoking for a long period of time. Is it fair to give new lungs to somebody because they chose to ruin their own?

Radiotherapy

During radiotherapy, concentrated waves of radiation are aimed at the tumour to try to shrink it. Small tumours can be treated this way instead of with surgery. Larger tumours can be prevented from growing bigger using radiotherapy.

The radiotherapy can either be administered as beams of radiation directed at the tumour from outside the body, or by placing a small piece of radioactive material directly next to the tumour using a very thin tube, called a catheter.

Chemotherapy

During chemotherapy, patients are injected with many different drugs. These either shrink the tumour before surgery, prevent the cancer from reoccurring, or provide relief from the symptoms of lung cancer when surgery is not possible.

Lung cancer patients are now more likely to be treated using a range of these strategies. For example, they might have surgery to remove the tumour and then have radiotherapy and chemotherapy to tackle any remaining cancerous cells.

Genetic research

It is not yet possible to use genetics to treat lung cancer.

However, scientists have been studying the genes of lung cancer sufferers in order to help doctors prescribe more effective treatments. For example, some chemotherapy drugs work better in lung cancer patients whose tumours have a certain genetic mutation.

The reason for this is not clear. However, it does show that treatment can be more effective if it is prescribed for the individual, rather than on a 'one size fits all' basis. This idea of tailoring treatments to a person's DNA is a growing field in medical research known as **pharmacogenomics**.

Prevention: the British government take action

The government was slow to respond to the evidence that cigarette smoking was linked to lung cancer. This evidence was first published in 1950. By 1985, smoking-related deaths cost the NHS £165 million a year. However, the government earned around £4 billion from the tobacco tax. There were thousands of jobs related to the tobacco industry in the UK. There was also an ethical issue: was it the government's job to limit personal freedoms?

However, as time passed, it became clear that the government needed to intervene. The death rate was too high – they would not normally ignore an epidemic of such magnitude.

This table shows some of the actions that the government took.

Changing behaviour The government passes laws to **force** people to change behaviour that damages their health.	Influencing behaviour The government controls communication to **influence** people to change behaviour that damages health.
In 2007, the government **banned smoking in all workplaces**. People were no longer allowed to smoke in pubs, cafés, restaurants or offices. In 2015, the **ban was extended to cars** carrying children under the age of 18. There is significant evidence to suggest that second-hand smoke has a negative impact on health, particularly among children. Although many still argue that a smoking ban is an attack on personal choice, others argue that it is not the choice of the child to be exposed to the smoke. Therefore, the government stepped in to protect their health.	The **ban on tobacco advertising** began with a ban on cigarette television advertising in 1965. Over time, the rules governing how and where cigarettes could be advertised were extended, until the government banned cigarette advertising entirely in 2005. This included the sponsorship of major sporting events in the UK, such as the Grand Prix.
In 2007, the government **raised the legal age for buying tobacco** from 16 to 18. They did this to try to reduce the number of teenagers who smoke.	The government has produced many **campaigns to advertise the dangers of smoking** over the past decades. These have included highlighting the impact of pregnant women smoking, the number of chemicals included in cigarette smoke and statistics about the health impacts and the diseases caused by regular use. Education to discourage young people from smoking is now included in schools.
Increased taxation on tobacco products was introduced to encourage people to stop smoking.	Government research in 2012 suggested that it is important to discourage young people from smoking. Now, all cigarette products in shops must be **removed from display**.

Source A

A 2012 Department of Health consultation on smoking, which sets out the reasons why the government has taken action to limit visibility of cigarettes.

Evidence shows that cigarette displays in shops can encourage young people to start smoking. The figures for England show that:

- 5% of children aged 11-15 are regular smokers
- more than 300,000 children under 16 try smoking each year
- 39% of smokers say that they were smoking regularly before the age of 16.

Covering tobacco displays will protect children and young people from the promotion of tobacco products in shops, helping them to resist the temptation to start smoking. It will also help and support adults who are trying to quit.

More than 8 million people in England still smoke – it is one of the biggest preventable killers causing more than 80,000 deaths each year. Nearly two-thirds of current and ex-smokers say they started smoking before they were 18.

Government campaigns and legislation have led to a change in attitude among the public. The number of smokers is falling. It is now very unlikely that you will see a television character or a public figure smoking. If you do, it will probably be portrayed negatively.

Case study comparison: government action against cholera vs government action against lung cancer

Government action	
Cholera	**Lung cancer**
Slow response initially. John Snow presented his findings about the link between dirty water and cholera in 1855, but a new sewer system took 20 years to be completed (and was not a direct response to Snow's findings).	**Slow response initially.** The first evidence linking smoking to lung cancer was published in 1950, but government did not directly intervene until death rates became too high to ignore.
More direct response in late 19th century. The 1875 Public Health Act forced cities to be cleaner to stop the spread of cholera, after more proof that Snow's findings were true.	**More direct response in early 21st century.** Government tried to both force and influence change in smoking behaviour. Smoking bans were introduced in 2007 and changes were made on how tobacco could be advertised.

Activities ?

1 Create a timeline to show the rise in lung cancer cases since c1900.

2 Explain how science and technology have changed the way lung cancer is diagnosed and treated.

3 Government action to combat lung cancer can be divided into three categories:

   a encouraging current smokers to quit

   b preventing people from becoming smokers

   c protecting non-smokers from the dangers of second-hand smoke.

4 Using the information above, divide the government actions among these categories. Has the government's focus changed over time?

Summary

- Lung cancer became a much more common disease after 1900.
- In 1950, scientists proved that smoking was linked to lung cancer.
- Lung cancer patients are diagnosed using a combination of scans and analysis of cells from the lung.
- Treatments including surgery, radiotherapy and chemotherapy have been developed. However, there is not yet a conclusive cure for lung cancer.
- Since the 1950s, the government has taken more action to combat smoking.

Checkpoint

Strengthen

S1 Which organisation published the 1950 study linking smoking with lung cancer?

S2 Name the methods by which lung cancer is diagnosed.

S3 Choose three government strategies aimed at preventing lung cancer and explain how they work.

Challenge

C1 How much has government intervention changed since c1900? Think back to previous periods to draw your comparison.

Before writing your answer, you might find it useful to create a mind map listing examples from each period you have studied.

Activity ?

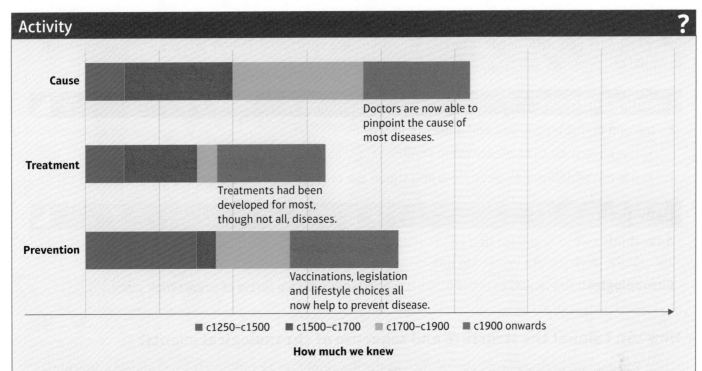

How much we knew

- ■ c1250–c1500
- ■ c1500–c1700
- ■ c1700–c1900
- ■ c1900 onwards

Cause: Doctors are now able to pinpoint the cause of most diseases.

Treatment: Treatments had been developed for most, though not all, diseases.

Prevention: Vaccinations, legislation and lifestyle choices all now help to prevent disease.

The progress table above shows the main areas of progress in this time period in **cause**, **treatment** and **prevention**. Using this table, make notes to explain why knowledge about cause, treatment and prevention of diseases was similar, c1900–present.

Recall quiz

1 Name the scientists who discovered the structure of DNA.
2 In what year was the human genome mapped?
3 What key piece of technology enabled the discovery of DNA?
4 When did the government pass the Clean Air Acts?
5 List three new methods of diagnosing patients since c1900.
6 Who developed the first two 'magic bullets' and what were they called?
7 What are the three strands of care available from the NHS?
8 Name two diseases that can now be prevented by immunisation.
9 Which key individuals were responsible for the discovery and development of penicillin?
10 Name three different treatments for lung cancer.

Activities ?

You've now completed your thematic study of medicine. It is a good time to look back over the whole time period and recap some of the things you have learned.

1 Draw a timeline from 1250 to 2000. Add onto it key information about ideas about the causes of disease and illness, methods of treatment and attempts at prevention. You could colour code these. Use the timeline on pages 10–11 to help you if you want.
2 In a group, discuss why the process of change speeded up so rapidly towards the end of the time period. Consider the impact of the key factors: individuals, institutions, science and technology, and attitudes in society.
3 When are the turning points in the history of medicine since 1250? You will need to create some criteria to help you to make this judgement.

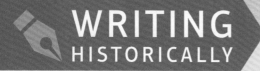

Writing historically: a well-structured response

Every response you write needs to be clearly written and structured. To help you achieve this, you need to signal the sequence and structure of your ideas clearly.

Learning outcomes

By the end of this lesson, you will understand how to:

- use adverbials to sequence events and developments chronologically
- use adverbials to link your ideas and signal the sequence and structure of your argument.

Definitions

Adverbial: a word or phrase that can modify a verb, adjective or another adverb, e.g. 'quickly', 'incredibly', 'such'; or can be used to link ideas, e.g 'similarly', 'consequently', 'therefore', etc.

Chronological: sequenced in order of time; the order in which a series of events took place.

How can I signal the structure and sequence of chronological events?

When you explain or describe a process, such as the development of antibiotics, you can use **adverbials** to signal the **chronological** order of events.

Look at this sequence of events describing the development of penicillin:

> The antibiotic, penicillin, was accidentally discovered by Alexander Fleming in 1928.
>
> Florey and Chain recognised its potential and began to refine the drug in 1939.
>
> The first human was treated with penicillin in 1944.
>
> Because of the Second World War, the drug was produced on an industrial scale from 1944.
>
> Fleming, Florey and Chain were awarded the Nobel Prize in 1945.

1. Write a paragraph about the development of penicillin, using some of the adverbials below to signal clearly and link the order of these events (note: adverbials don't always need to go at the start of the sentence, e.g. 'The first human was eventually treated with penicillin in 1944').

> Firstly... Secondly... Then... Soon... Next... Meanwhile... Eventually... Finally...

2. You could use a wider range of adverbials to signal much more clearly and precisely the timescale over which penicillin was developed. Look at the examples below. Use them to help you rewrite your paragraph, making it as clear and precise as possible.

> Initially... Previously... Before... During... After several years... Within three years...
>
> Eleven years later... In the following year... By 1944... From 1939 to 1945...

3. Compare your answers to Questions 1 and 2. Which version do you prefer? Write a sentence or two explaining your decision.

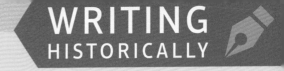
How can I signal the structure and sequence of my argument?

You can use adverbials to link your ideas and guide the reader through your argument. For example:

Similarly... For example... Such as... However... Therefore... Consequently...

Moreover... Nonetheless... Furthermore... On the other hand... In addition... Above all...

Significantly... In conclusion...

4. Now look at the two extracts below from a response to the following exam-style question. Make a note of all the adverbials the writer used to link their ideas and structure their argument.

'The greatest factor on the advancement of the treatment of disease between 1700–1900 was science and technology'. How far do you agree? **(20 marks)**

For most of the 19th century, doctors could do little to treat specific diseases. Consequently, traditional approaches such as bleeding remained common. However, the science of chemistry improved in the second half of the 19th century and French chemist, Louis Pasteur, proved germ theory – that specific bacteria caused specific diseases, such as anthrax.

Science and technology were, therefore, a key factor in the improvements in medical treatment. There are, on the other hand, other factors to consider.

5. Adverbials can show different kinds of connections. Look at the adverbials at the top of this page. Make a copy of the table and write them in the right category.

Causation and consequence	
Addition	
Contrast	
Exemplification	
Emphasis	

Did you notice?

Adverbials can be positioned at a number of different points in a sentence.

6. At what point in the sentences above are most of the adverbials positioned?

7. Choose one sentence from the response above in which an adverbial is used. Experiment with repositioning the adverbial at different points in the sentence. What impact does it have on the clarity of the sentence?

Improving an answer

Now look at the final paragraph below, which is a response to the exam-style question above.

Both of these factors are interdependent and important. The scientific and technological breakthroughs of the 19th and 20th centuries (x-rays, antibiotics, radiotherapy) were the more fundamental. The funding of the NHS by government had a huge impact on people's access to healthcare. Without the breakthroughs this would have had considerably less impact.

8. Rewrite this conclusion using a range of adverbials to signal the development of the argument clearly.

Preparing for your GCSE Paper 1 exam

Paper 1 overview

Paper 1 is in two sections that examine the Historic Environment and the Thematic Study. Together they count for 30% of your History assessment. The questions on the Thematic Study: 'Medicine through time' are in Section B and are worth 20% of your History assessment. Allow two-thirds of the examination time for Section B. There are an extra four marks for the assessment of Spelling, Punctuation and Grammar in the last question.

History Paper 1	Historic Environment and Thematic Depth Study			Time 1 hour 15 mins
Section A	Historic Environment	Answer 3 questions	16 marks	25 mins
Section B	Thematic Study	Answer 3 questions	32 marks + 4 SPaG marks	50 mins

Medicine through time, c1250-present

You need to answer Questions 3 and 4, and then **either** Question 5 or Question 6.

Q3 Explain one way... (4 marks)

You are given about half a page of lines to write about a similarity or a difference. Allow five minutes to write your answer. This question is only worth four marks and you should keep the answer brief. Only one comparison is needed. You should compare by referring to both periods given in the question – for example, 'xxx was similar, because in the Middle Ages… and also in the 16th century…'

Q4 Explain why... (12 marks)

This question asks you to explain the reasons why something happened. Allow about 15 minutes to write your answer. You are given two information points as prompts to help you. You do not have to use the prompts and you will not lose marks by leaving them out. Higher marks are gained by adding in a point extra to the prompts. You will be given at least two pages of lines in the answer booklet for your answer. This does not mean you should try to fill all the space. The front page of the exam paper states 'there may be more space than you need'. Aim to write an answer giving at least three explained reasons.

EITHER Q5 OR Q6 How far do you agree? (16 marks +4 for SPaG)

This question is worth 20 marks, including SPaG – more than half your marks for the whole of the Thematic Study. Make sure to keep 30 minutes of the exam time to answer it and to check your spelling, punctuation and grammar. You will have prompts to help, as for Question 4. You have a choice of questions: Q5 or Q6. Before you decide, be clear what the statement is about and what topic information will you need to answer it. The statement may be about one of the following concepts: significance, cause, consequence, change, continuity, similarity, difference. It is a good idea during revision to practise identifying the concept focus of statements. You could do this with everyday examples and test one another: 'The bus was late because it broke down' = statement about cause; 'The bus broke down as a result of poor maintenance' = statement about consequence. 'The bus service has improved recently' = statement about change.

You must make a judgement and you should think about both sides of the argument. Plan your answer before you begin to write, putting your points under two headings: For and Against. You should consider at least three points. Think of each point as adding weight to one side of the argument or the other. Even if you make some points against the statement, if the 'For' side ends up with more weight, the judgement in your conclusion should be that you agree with the statement. This will give you a coherent answer that hangs together. Be clear about your reasons (criteria) for your judgement – for example, why is one cause more important than another? Did it perhaps set others in motion?

In this question, four extra marks will be gained for good spelling, punctuation and grammar. Use sentences, paragraphs, capital letters, commas and full stops, etc. Try also to use specialist terms specific to your Thematic Study – for example about society in the Middle Ages or the use of technology in the 20th century.

On the one hand
- *Point 1*

On the other hand
- *Point 2*
- *Point 3*

Conclusion

130

Paper 1, Question 3

Explain **one** way in which ideas about the treatment of disease were different in the 17th century from ideas in the 13th century. **(4 marks)**

Exam tip

This answer should not be very long, but it does need to have specific information for each period. Try to identify a difference between the two periods, and then give a specific example for each one.

Average answer

Herbal remedies such as mint and camomile were very common. Then there were more chemical cures, although they still used herbal remedies as well.

This answer identifies treatments in each period. There is some recognition of difference by using the word 'then'. The answer does not specify periods, so is vague. It lacks supporting examples.

Verdict

This is an average answer because the candidate has provided general comments about the difference in treatment between the two periods.
Use the feedback to rewrite this answer, making as many improvements as you can.

Strong answer

In the 13th century, many people were treated with herbal remedies. These were usually made with local plants and herbs such as mint and camomile. Recipes for these included theriaca, a popular remedy.
Although herbal remedies were still used in the 17th century, more materials were available due to increased overseas trading. New ingredients included nutmeg and cinnamon. There were also experiments with chemical cures, for example, the use of mercury to treat syphilis.

This answer describes treatments in both centuries. It gives specific examples of treatments used and explains what the difference is and what caused it, using the wider context of trade.

Verdict

This is a strong answer because it features specific information about the topic to demonstrate the difference in treatments.

Paper 1, Question 4

Explain why there was rapid change in the prevention of smallpox in the period c1750–c1900.

You may use the following information in your answer:
- inoculation
- Edward Jenner.

You **must** also use information of your own.　　　**(12 marks)**

Exam tip

Make sure you bring in your own knowledge as well as what is suggested by the bullet points. If you don't, you are limiting yourself to a maximum of eight marks.

Average answer

Before 1798, people used to inoculate themselves against smallpox. They did this by making a cut in their arm and rubbing in pus from a person with a mild case of smallpox. This sometimes worked.

In 1797, Edward Jenner realised that people who had had cowpox didn't catch smallpox. He carried out an experiment where he rubbed the pus from a cowpox sufferer into a cut on the arm of a boy. He became immune to smallpox. Jenner called this a vaccination, after the Latin word for cow.

After that the government were keen to give Jenner funding to develop the vaccination and they made it compulsory. Due to this, lots of people in Britain started to get the smallpox vaccination and this prevented the disease from spreading. By 1979 smallpox had been eradicated from the world.

Therefore there was rapid change in the prevention of smallpox after 1798 because Jenner invented the vaccination and the government made it the law that people had to have it.

There is a good spread of knowledge. The factors of individuals and institutions (the government) have been expressed, though not directly. The style is quite narrative. Points should be more closely linked to the question. There is a clear chronological structure.

Verdict

This is an average answer because:
- there is a good focus on the conceptual focus of the question (rapid change in prevention of smallpox) but this needs to be more explicit.
- there is accurate and relevant information but it is not precisely selected – some of it is not useful in explaining the reasons for rapid change.

Use the feedback to rewrite this answer, making as many improvements as you can.

Paper 1, Question 4

Explain why there was rapid change in the prevention of smallpox in the period c1750–c1900. **(12 marks)**

Strong answer

Change occurred rapidly between c1750 and c1900 because of an individual – Edward Jenner – and an institution – the government.

Before 1798, people attempted to prevent smallpox using inoculation. This was not a trustworthy method, as many of those who were infected with the smallpox virus died from the disease. Edward Jenner developed the world's first vaccination between 1797 and 1799, using material from sufferers of cowpox. He had observed that people who suffered from cowpox were immune to smallpox and used experiments to prove that this method worked. This was a big change in the ability to prevent smallpox.

However, Jenner's vaccination was not immediately popular due to attitudes in society. People did not trust the new method because he could not prove it with science. Many people, including inoculators and the Church, were against it. This meant that Jenner was only responsible for the rapid change in understanding how smallpox could be prevented.

It was the influence of the government that enabled the change to occur rapidly. From the start of the 19th century the government funded and encouraged vaccination programmes. For example, in 1807 they asked the Royal College of Physicians to organise vaccination nationwide and in 1852 they made the vaccination compulsory. Some historians argue that the big change occurred after 1867, when the vaccination was properly enforced.

Therefore, the change in understanding of how to prevent smallpox occurred when Jenner invented the vaccination; however, this did not become a rapid change until the government backed its use from the middle of the 19th century. Deaths from smallpox fell by approximately 85% between 1850 and 1880. This shows that the vaccination was successful in preventing outbreaks.

This answer is consistently analytical with a clear focus on the question throughout. Information is precisely selected to support the points made. There is a clear line of reasoning. The candidate has chosen to address the question directly in the conclusion, distinguishing between change and rapid change and making a judgement about the most important factor, although this is not actually required.

Verdict

This is a good answer because:

- it has included only relevant information
- the line of reasoning is consistently developed throughout the answer, with a strong focus on the factors
- there is a concluding paragraph that sums up the precise cause of rapid change.

Paper 1, Question 5/6

'The Theory of the Four Humours was the main idea about the cause of disease in the Middle Ages.'

How far do you agree? Explain your answer. You may use the following information in your answer:

- university training
- Galen's ideas.

You **must** also use some information of your own.

(16 marks + 4 for SPaG)

Average answer

During the Middle Ages, the Theory of the Four Humours was the main idea about the cause of disease. This theory had been created in ancient Greece by Hippocrates and developed by Galen in the Roman Empire. It was preferred by the medieval church because the theory suggested that the body was perfectly designed and this fitted with their ideas about man being made in God's image.

The theory said that people got ill because their humours were unbalanced. The four humours were blood, phlegm, black bile and yellow bile. An imbalance in one meant that a person would become ill. For example, a person suffering from a fever had too much blood. The treatment for this was eating something cool, like cucumber, and being bled, either by cutting into the body and draining blood or using a more gentle method, like leeches. Leeches were often used for old or young patients.

The Theory of the Four Humours was mainly used by physicians when diagnosing illnesses. This was because the Church was responsible for training doctors and they taught the works of Galen.

There were some other ideas about the causes of disease in the Middle Ages. For example, some people believed that God sent disease as a punishment for sin, particularly after the Black Death arrived in Britain in 1348. However, before 1348 most people believed in the Theory of the Four Humours because that's what doctors used.

Accurate information is given, although this is sometimes irrelevant, for example the explanation of treatments based on the humours. There is some analysis with reference to the question, although this is not sustained throughout. Some criteria have been provided for the judgement (early and late Middle Ages) but these are not developed.

Verdict

This is an average answer because:

- it includes specific, valid information, although some of this is poorly selected
- there is an explanation, showing some analysis of the question, particularly in the conclusion; however this is not consistent throughout
- the overall judgement has some justification but this needs to be more explicit.

Use the feedback to rewrite this answer, making as many improvements as you can.

Paper 1, Question 5/6

'The Theory of the Four Humours was the main idea about the cause of disease in the Middle Ages'.
How far do you agree? Explain your answer.　　**(16 marks + 4 for SPaG)**

Strong answer

To be judged as the main idea about the cause of disease in the Middle Ages, the theory in question should have been widely-known and popular throughout the whole time period.

The Theory of the Four Humours was promoted by the Church as an explanation of the cause of disease in the Middle Ages. They liked the theory because it fitted with the Bible's idea that man is designed in God's image. Therefore, the theory was taught to physicians in universities and this meant that they referred to the theory when diagnosing patients. Therefore, in terms of widely-known theories, this was the main one.

The theory suggested that disease was caused by an imbalance in the humours. These were linked to the seasons and, later, the positions of the planets. The theory was very popular because it could be twisted to explain practically any disease. People understood the theory and believed it to be true. Therefore, in terms of staying power, this theory was the main one, because it lasted all the way up until the 17th century.

However, the theory was not the only explanation for diseases in the Middle Ages. Many people also believed that God was responsible. God sent disease as a test for the devout, or to punish sin. A good example of this is during the outbreak of the Black Death in 1348. Many people believed that God had sent the disease as a punishment for their sins.

Other people believed that disease was caused by evil vapours, or miasma, that were present in the air and spread disease. Dirt and rotting matter were responsible for spreading the miasmata and breathing it in led to disease. Some people also believed that earthquakes or volcanos released disease-carrying miasma.

However, it is important to note that people who believed God sent disease also believed in the theory: God created an imbalance in the humours, which caused the disease. The same is true about the idea of a miasma causing disease: people believed that inhaling a miasma upset the balance of the humours.

Therefore, in terms of popularity, it could be argued that the theory was the main idea about the cause of disease in the Middle Ages, because even people who believed other theories followed it.

> There is a clear focus on the question from the outset, with criteria for making the judgement set out at the start and referred to throughout. The evidence selected to support the analysis shows an exceptional grasp of the wider context of the Middle Ages. Points are carefully linked to ensure the answer does not contradict itself at any point.

Verdict

This is a good answer because:

- there is a consistently analytical focus, backed by very precise knowledge
- criteria for reaching the judgement have been set out and applied throughout
- there is a clear line of reasoning running through the answer.

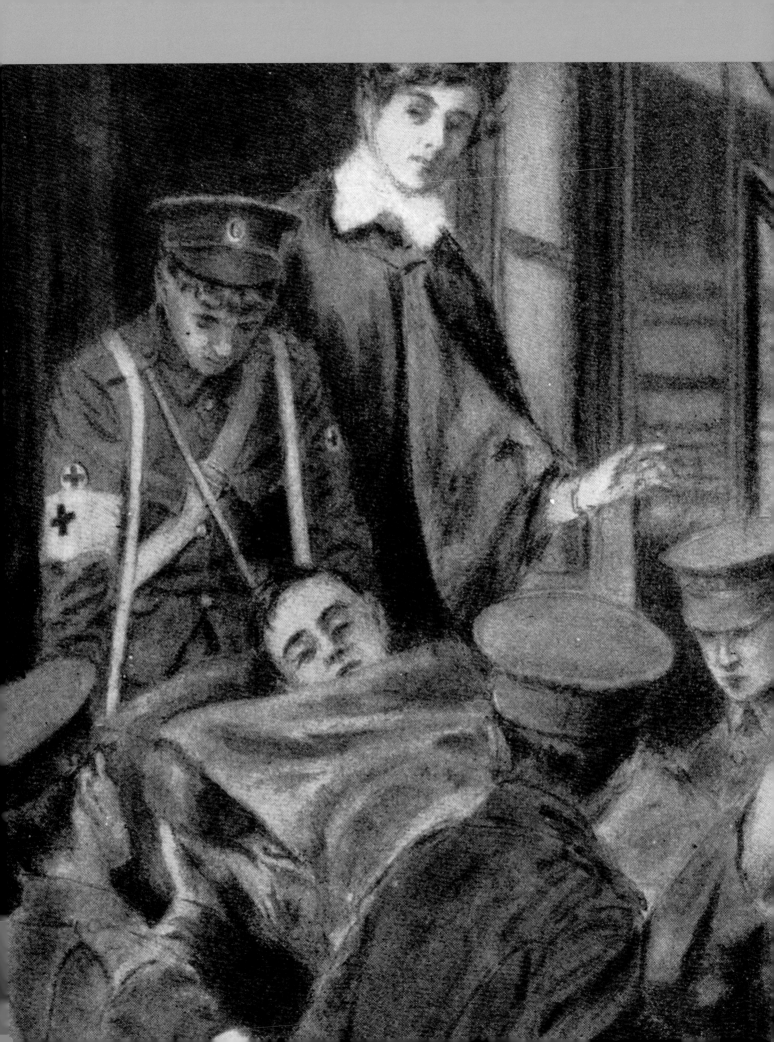

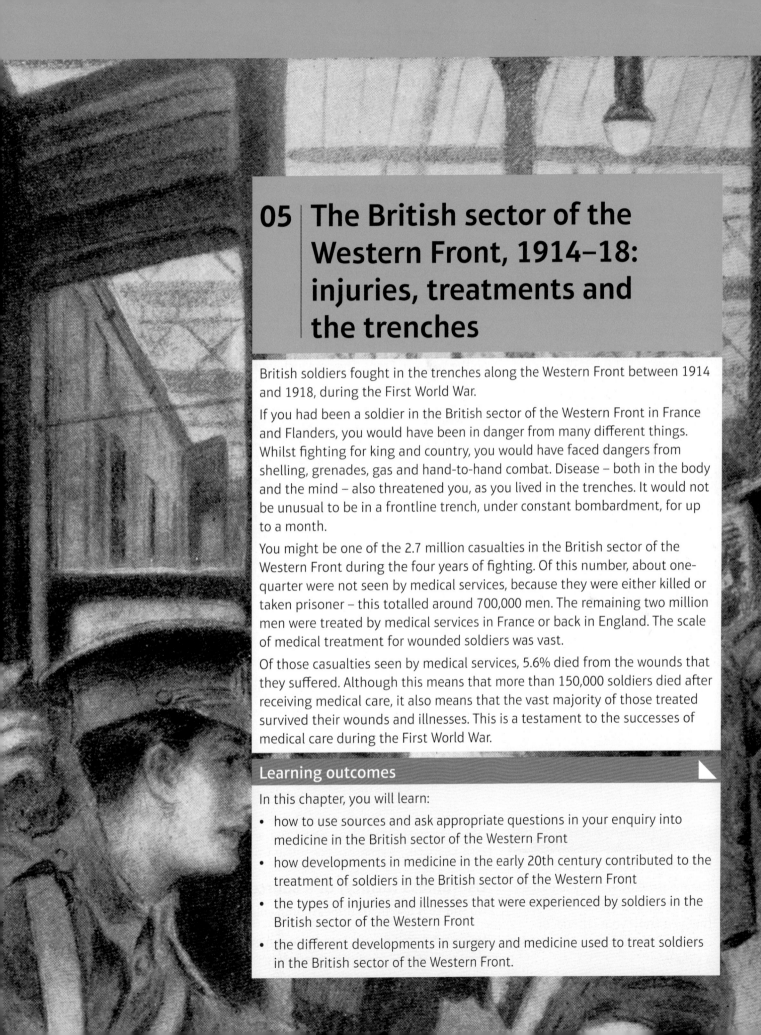

05 | The British sector of the Western Front, 1914–18: injuries, treatments and the trenches

British soldiers fought in the trenches along the Western Front between 1914 and 1918, during the First World War.

If you had been a soldier in the British sector of the Western Front in France and Flanders, you would have been in danger from many different things. Whilst fighting for king and country, you would have faced dangers from shelling, grenades, gas and hand-to-hand combat. Disease – both in the body and the mind – also threatened you, as you lived in the trenches. It would not be unusual to be in a frontline trench, under constant bombardment, for up to a month.

You might be one of the 2.7 million casualties in the British sector of the Western Front during the four years of fighting. Of this number, about one-quarter were not seen by medical services, because they were either killed or taken prisoner – this totalled around 700,000 men. The remaining two million men were treated by medical services in France or back in England. The scale of medical treatment for wounded soldiers was vast.

Of those casualties seen by medical services, 5.6% died from the wounds that they suffered. Although this means that more than 150,000 soldiers died after receiving medical care, it also means that the vast majority of those treated survived their wounds and illnesses. This is a testament to the successes of medical care during the First World War.

Learning outcomes

In this chapter, you will learn:

- how to use sources and ask appropriate questions in your enquiry into medicine in the British sector of the Western Front
- how developments in medicine in the early 20th century contributed to the treatment of soldiers in the British sector of the Western Front
- the types of injuries and illnesses that were experienced by soldiers in the British sector of the Western Front
- the different developments in surgery and medicine used to treat soldiers in the British sector of the Western Front.

Sources and the examination

Source A

From an interview with Gunner William Towers in 1989. Here, he is recalling his treatment following a wound to his leg at Ypres in October 1917.

They took us to a hospital at Étaples and fitted me with a Thomas splint, a round wooden ring with iron bands and a footrest. The pain from my knee was getting terrible so when I saw an officer coming up with his arm around two sisters and laughing, I said, 'Excuse me, Sir, could you have a look at my knee?' He came over and he stank of whisky. When the nurses took the bandages off he said, 'Oh there's fluid above the knee. We'll tap that tonight.' So they came for me to go to the theatre and I thought, 'Thank God for that.' But when I woke up in the early hours of the morning I thought, 'Oh my God. My leg's gone.' They'd guillotined it off without saying a word. There had been no hint at all that I was going to lose my leg. They hadn't even looked at it until I asked the doctor.

After that they put me on a boat and I was taken to England. A civilian doctor came to look at me and when he took the bandages off the smell was terrible. He thought I was going to die.

Key term

Criteria*

The measure by which you judge something. It is vital in History that you know your criteria, or criterion (singular) before judging a source.

In the examination you will be given **two** sources, and you are asked to do **two** things with these sources:

- comment on the **usefulness of both** sources for an enquiry
- write about **a detail in one source** that you would **follow up**, the new question this detail prompts you to ask, the type of source you would want to answer your new question and why that source might help you answer your new question.

Because most of the marks in this section of the examination are for your work with sources, there are more sources in this chapter than the rest of the book. Source A is about the Third Battle of Ypres. Source B is about the Battle of the Somme. The Battle of the Somme was one of the most challenging battles for the medical services to deal with because of the high casualty rate. Sources A and B are both examples of records of medical work on the Western Front. They are included to help you understand how the examination works.

Source B

From Pat Beauchamp's autobiography, *Fanny Goes to War*, published in 1919. Beauchamp first worked as a nurse, bringing in the wounded from the trenches, and from 1916 as an ambulance driver. Here she is describing driving casualties to the Base Hospitals.

The battle of the Somme was in progress. Besides barges and day trains, three ambulance trains arrived each week. The whole Convoy turned out for this; and one by one the twenty-five odd cars would set off, keeping an equal distance apart, forming an imposing looking column down from the camp, across the bridge and through the town to the railway siding... Arrived at the big railway siding, we all formed up into a straight line to await the train... The ambulances were then reversed right up to the doors, and the stretcher bearers soon filled them up with four lying cases [wounded who could not walk]... Those journeys back were perfect nightmares. Try as one would, it was impossible not to bump a certain amount over those appalling roads full of holes and cobbles. It was pathetic when a voice from the interior could be heard asking, "Is it much farther, Sister?" and knowing how far it was, my heart ached for them. After all they had been through, one felt they should be spared every extra bit of pain that was possible. When I in my turn was in an ambulance, I knew just what it felt like. Sometimes the cases were so bad we feared they would not even last the journey, and there we were all alone, and not able to hurry to hospital owing to the other three on board.

Usefulness (utility) of a source

No source is useful (or useless) until you have an enquiry. Our enquiry is:

How useful are Sources A and B for an enquiry into the problems that faced the medical services during battles on the Western Front? To answer this question you will need to explain the criteria* for your judgement.

They might be based on your analysis of:

- the content of the source – what does it tell you?
- the nature, origin, and purpose of the source
- the context of the source – how fitting it into what you already know about the problems that faced the medical services helps you understand the source better – you might comment on its accuracy, selectiveness, or typicality.

How does this work in practice?

- Source A is a person remembering events that happened about 70 years previously. William Towers provides us with a description of traumatic events that he has experienced, and these would stick in his mind. This would support your criterion for saying it could be useful because it is **likely** to be true. This shows you have thought about the actual source, rather than just saying it is 70 years later so he may have misremembered. You could say that about any source that relies on memory, and it really depends on what people are trying to remember.
- Source B tells us that the wounded were transported by ambulance from the ambulance trains to the Base Hospitals. More interestingly, it tells us about the personal reaction of one ambulance driver to the job she was doing. This might be the best to use as a criteria for judging the usefulness of the source – it tells us something unusual and relevant.

- When you've studied this topic a bit more, you could show how this source fits into your knowledge by pointing out that Casualty Clearing Stations and Base Hospitals were stages in the chain of evacuation of soldiers from the frontline.

You will use the criteria to build your answer. The best answers will use criteria drawn from all the three possible areas:

- content
- provenance (nature, origin and purpose)
- context (how it fits into what you already know).

Following up on sources

Where possible, historians try to use as many different types of source as they can. There is a good reason for this. Each different type of source has different strengths and weaknesses. Figure 5.1 shows the range of different types of source a historian can use.

The second question about sources asks you to pick a detail from one of the sources, and then you will explain how you would follow that detail up in a different type of source. It makes more sense to think about that when you know a bit more about the range of sources, so we will come back to that later.

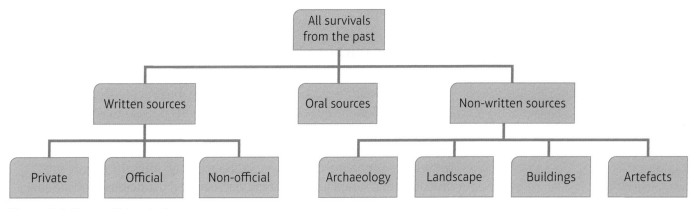

Figure 5.1 Types of historical sources.

Activities ?

1 In small groups, study Source C and make a list of criteria you could use to judge its usefulness.

2 Using the categories from Figure 5.1, make a list of sources that could be used to study your own life.

 a Give at least one example source in each category.

 b Explain why each example would be useful.

3 Your enquiry is 'the problems that faced the medical services during the Battle of the Somme'.

 a Copy Figure 5.1, leaving lots of space in the boxes on the lowest row.

 b Look ahead at the sources in the rest of this chapter, and list in the boxes on your diagram one example of each type of source that could be used for your enquiry into the problems that faced the medical services during the Battle of the Somme.

Source C

Photograph of a wounded British soldier being carried on a stretcher by German prisoners of war, 15 September 1916. This followed a battle that was part of the Somme campaign.

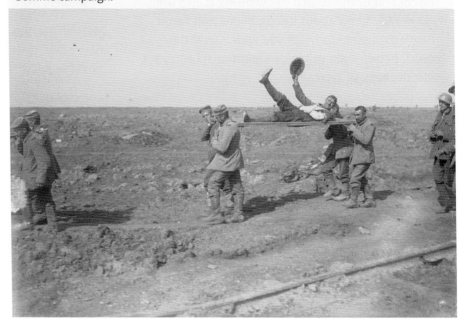

Provenance

Historians think very carefully about their sources. They test them to check whether they are really appropriate for the way they want to use them. The tests are:

- what is its purpose?
- what is the standpoint of the author or artist?
- is it part of the action or reflecting on the action?

What is its purpose?

When, where, and why was the source created and who by? When we read something about the problems that faced the medical services during the Battle of the Somme by someone who was there, it helps to know if they wrote this at the time or many years later. Just because it was written at the time does not mean it is true. A nurse driving an ambulance might have written to her parents back home a couple of days after the events she describes. She would likely not tell them in detail the deaths that she saw. In this case, the purpose of the source might be to keep in contact with her parents, rather than to tell the whole truth about what she was doing.

What is the standpoint of the author or artist?

This can grow out of thinking about provenance. Does the person have a particular point of view? If you are reading a description of the medical treatment received by soldiers during the Battle of the Somme, it might be useful to know whether it was written by an opponent or a supporter of the government. For example, government propaganda was deliberately created to change people's views. It might be exaggerated, it might leave things out or it might just not be true. This doesn't mean historians don't use propaganda – it provides much useful evidence, but its use might be revealing what the government wanted people to believe, rather than what really happened.

Is it part of the action or reflecting on the action?

What is the difference between a live radio commentary on a football match, and the account of that same game written years later in a player's autobiography? Both have their strengths, but they are very different.

Turning a source into evidence

A source is only useful, and it can only be turned into evidence, when you have a question or enquiry. For example, Source B isn't either useful or not useful in itself. If we have an enquiry of either: a) the role of ambulance drivers in driving the wounded to Base Hospitals, or b) conditions in the Casualty Clearing Stations, then we can think about whether it is useful or not. In the case of enquiry a) it is useful, and in the case of enquiry b) it isn't.

Judging sources

- Start with the provenance (the nature, origin and purpose of the source). Does this suggest strengths or weaknesses when using this source? For example, we don't know if Source C was taken as propaganda to reassure people that things were going well. Could it have been staged?

- Move on to content usefulness. What can you learn from the source that is relevant? What can you work out from it? Does it tell you new things, adding to your understanding?

- It is easier to use photos as sources if we know **why** they were taken. Often, we don't. The best you can do is think carefully about the context and content of the photograph.

THINKING HISTORICALLY Evidence (2a)

Information and evidence

Information only becomes evidence when we use it **to work out** something about an issue in the past. Information needs to be questioned before we can use it as **evidence** to draw conclusions. Without a question, information doesn't tell us very much.

Study the following questions about the Western Front:

1 How was medical treatment at the frontline carried out?	2 Why did trench warfare begin?	3 What were the main battles?
4 What sort of injuries did the soldiers receive?	5 What did people in Britain think about the Western Front?	6 Where were the medical facilities located?

Study Sources A, B, and C.

1 Which of the six questions would the sources **not** help us answer?

2 Which question is Source A most useful in providing evidence for?

Look at Source C. Draw up a table with three columns labelled 'Question', 'Inference' and 'Evidence'.

3 Write out Question 1 in the first column. Then use Source C to fill in the other two columns with inferences you can make that answer the question, and evidence from the source that backs up each inference.

4 Write out Question 5 in a new row, and add inferences and evidence for this question from Source C.

5 Look at the inferences you've made from Source C. Are they the same for both questions?

6 Write a new question that you could use Source C to help answer.

7 In your own words, explain how the question you ask affects what evidence you find in a source.

In the years before the outbreak of the First World War, many medical breakthroughs had occurred. These were used as the foundation for medical advancements in the British sector of the Western Front. These included aseptic surgery, x-rays and blood transfusions.

Understanding infection and the move towards aseptic surgery

Joseph Lister first used carbolic acid to prevent infection in surgery in 1865, based on Louis Pasteur's work on Germ Theory.

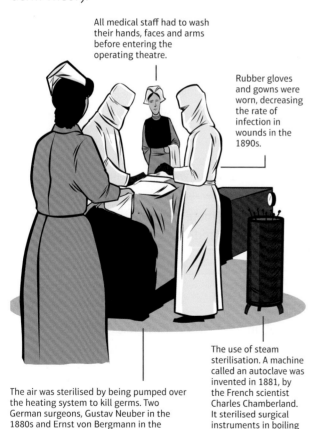

All medical staff had to wash their hands, faces and arms before entering the operating theatre.

Rubber gloves and gowns were worn, decreasing the rate of infection in wounds in the 1890s.

The use of steam sterilisation. A machine called an autoclave was invented in 1881, by the French scientist Charles Chamberland. It sterilised surgical instruments in boiling steam.

The air was sterilised by being pumped over the heating system to kill germs. Two German surgeons, Gustav Neuber in the 1880s and Ernst von Bergmann in the 1890s, first developed these methods.

Figure 5.2 The key features of early 20th-century aseptic surgery.

By the late 1890s, Lister's methods had laid the foundations for aseptic surgery. By 1900, most operations were carried out using aseptic methods.

The development of x-rays

The development of x-rays was completely accidental. In 1895, Wilhelm Roentgen, a German physicist, was studying the effects of passing an electrical current through a glass tube covered in black paper. He noticed that although everything in the room was darkened, a screen about a metre from the equipment had begun to glow. He called these rays that could pass through glass 'x'.

Further experiments led him to realise that these rays could penetrate many objects. He held a piece of lead in front of the tube and was able to see his own flesh glowing around his bones. He then placed photographic paper between the tube and his hand and created the world's first x-ray image. Shortly after, he also took an x-ray of his wife's left hand. It was possible to see not just her hand on this x-ray, but also her wedding ring.

The importance of the use of x-rays was understood immediately.

As early as 1896, radiology departments* were opening in a number of British hospitals, contributing to advancing knowledge and applying the new science in a medical setting. At Glasgow Royal Infirmary, a radiology department headed by Dr John Macintyre produced a number of interesting x-rays, including x-rays of a kidney stone, a penny in a child's throat, and even a frog's legs in motion.

At Birmingham General Hospital, Dr John Hall-Edwards was one of the first doctors to make a diagnosis based on information from an x-ray, when he located a needle in a woman's hand. It was this potential for carrying out diagnosis before operations took place that would help medical treatments on the Western Front.

However, many problems emerged with the early use of x-rays.

- The health risks associated with x-rays were not fully understood. The amount of radiation that was released in early x-rays was about 1,500 times the amount that is released today. Exposure to x-rays was harmful. Patients could lose hair or suffer burns.
- Wilhelm Roentgen had used a table-top machine, but the glass tube used with this was very fragile, so could break easily.
- Taking an x-ray of a hand using the table-top machine took about 90 minutes – which was a very long time to keep your hand still!
- Larger x-ray machines were being developed, but were very difficult to move around.

However, these dangers and problems did not prevent the continuing use of x-rays.

> **Key term**
>
> **Radiology department***
> The hospital department where x-rays are carried out.

Source A

A 19th-century x-ray machine in a hospital.

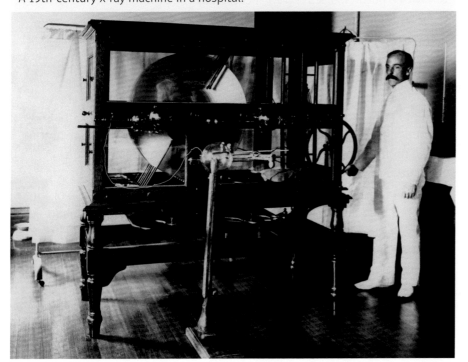

> **Activities**   **?**
>
> Look at Source A.
>
> 1 Describe the main features of the machine shown.
>
> 2 What problems might arise from the use of this machine?
>
> 3 What other types of sources might help you to understand the problems linked to the use of x-rays?

Key terms

Blood transfusion*

Blood taken from a healthy person and given to another person.

Universal blood group*

This blood group can be used in a transfusion to a recipient with any other blood group.

The development of blood transfusions and the storage of blood

An average adult body contains about five litres of blood. If somebody loses too much blood, then they are likely to go into shock and die. In the 19th and early 20th centuries, blood loss was often the result of complex surgeries.

With the development of aseptic surgery and x-rays in the late 19th century, it was possible to carry out more complex surgical operations safely. However, if the problem of blood loss could not be solved, then the success of these operations would be irrelevant.

James Blundell did the first experiments in human blood transfusion* in 1818 to help women under his medical care who lost blood when they gave birth. Between 1818 and 1829, Blundell carried out ten transfusions, with up to half of the patients surviving. In these years, Blundell developed many of the techniques and basic equipment which would continue to be used up to the First World War. As blood could not be stored – it had to be used as soon as it was available – transfusions were carried out with the donor (the person giving the blood) being directly connected to the recipient (the person receiving the blood) by a tube.

The table below shows the main problems with blood transfusions, and the attempts that had been made to solve them by the early 20th century.

Activities ?

1. What were the main features of aseptic surgery?
2. Do you think that the benefits of x-rays outweighed their dangers?
3. With a partner, discuss how successfully the problems associated with blood transfusions had been solved by the early 20th century.

Problem with transfusion	Attempted solution to the problem
Blood coagulates (clots) as soon as it leaves the body. This meant that the tubes which transfused blood from one person to another could become blocked up.	There were attempts to find chemicals, such as sodium bicarbonate, to prevent clotting. In 1894, Professor Almroth Wright, a British scientist, concluded that the soluble solution of certain acids could prevent clotting, but he thought that side effects, such as convulsions, could not be prevented.
Rejection of the transfused blood because the blood of the donor and the blood of the recipient was not compatible.	In 1901, Austrian doctor Karl Landsteiner discovered the existence of three different blood groups – A, B and O. The following year a fourth blood group, AB, was also found. This information was used in 1907 by Reuben Ottenberg, an American doctor, who was the first person to match a donor and a recipient's blood type before a transfusion. He also identified blood group O as a universal blood group.*
Danger of infection from unsterilised equipment.	The introduction of aseptic methods of surgery had largely solved this problem in hospital conditions by the early 20th century.

Summary

- By 1900, most surgery was carried out using aseptic methods.
- X-rays were discovered in 1895. They were used almost immediately for diagnostic purposes in medicine.
- Blood transfusions had to take place on a person-to-person basis because there was no way to store blood.
- The recognition of different blood groups enabled blood transfusions to become more effective.

Checkpoint

Strengthen

S1 Explain how the following were important developments in medicine?

- Aseptic surgery
- X-rays
- Blood transfusions

Challenge

C1 Although there had been many advances in medicine, there were still many problems remaining. Identify these problems.

C2 From your list of problems, which ones do you think would be particularly challenging in a war environment?

If you are not confident about any of these questions, form a group with other students, discuss the answers and then record your conclusions. Your teacher can give you some hints.

Flanders and northern France

Britain declared war on Germany on August 4 1914. Germany invaded France through Belgium. The British government sent the British Expeditionary Force (BEF) to northern France to try to stop the German advance through Belgium. The BEF was made up of 70,000 professional soldiers, fighting alongside a larger French army. Near Mons, close to the French-Belgian border, the BEF faced a German army that was more than double their size – 160,000 soldiers. Although they stopped the German advance briefly, they were ordered to retreat to the River Marne in order to prevent Paris falling to the Germans. After the Battle of the Marne, the German forces pulled back to the River Aisne and it was here that trench warfare began.

The trench system

By the end of 1914, much of Belgium and northern France had been occupied by the Germans, although they had been stopped from advancing into the heart of France. This meant that battles could not follow along the same lines as previous wars, which had involved much more movement of single armies. Instead, it became a static war based on trenches, which needed to be defended from the enemy, with attempts made to advance from the trenches to seize land from the enemy army. A line of trenches was eventually established all the way from the English Channel in the north, to Switzerland in the south.

Construction and organisation

Although some basic trenches were dug in 1914, a more complex system began to evolve from 1915. The trenches were generally dug to a depth of about 2.5 m. The main elements in the trench system are shown in Figure 5.3.

Trenches were easier to defend than attack. Machine guns could fire rapidly, and barbed wire was placed in **no-man's-land** (the area between two opposing lines of trenches) to slow down the progress of any attack.

New tactics were developed to try to deal with the advantages held by the defenders. Such tactics included the use of gas.

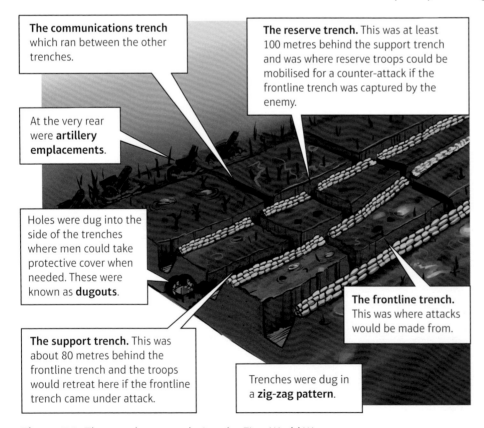

The communications trench which ran between the other trenches.

The reserve trench. This was at least 100 metres behind the support trench and was where reserve troops could be mobilised for a counter-attack if the frontline trench was captured by the enemy.

At the very rear were **artillery emplacements**.

Holes were dug into the side of the trenches where men could take protective cover when needed. These were known as **dugouts**.

The support trench. This was about 80 metres behind the frontline trench and the troops would retreat here if the frontline trench came under attack.

Trenches were dug in a **zig-zag pattern**.

The frontline trench. This was where attacks would be made from.

Figure 5.3 The trench system during the First World War.

Source A

A typical trench system, sketched during the war. The exact date and artist is not known. It was likely sketched after 1915.

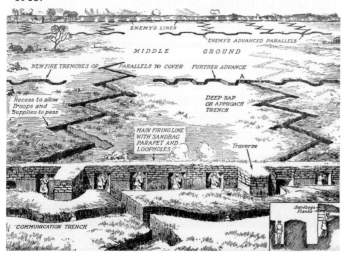

Source B

A British trench during the Battle of the Somme, July 1916.

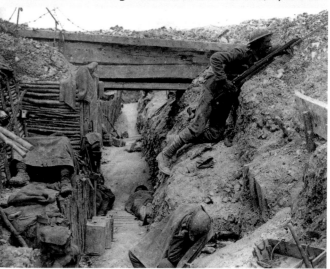

Activities ?

Study Sources A and B.

1 What differences do you note between the sketch diagram of a trench system and the photo of a trench?

2 What are the benefits and drawbacks of each of these types of sources for the historian?

3 Work in pairs. Discuss which of the two sources you find the most helpful and why.

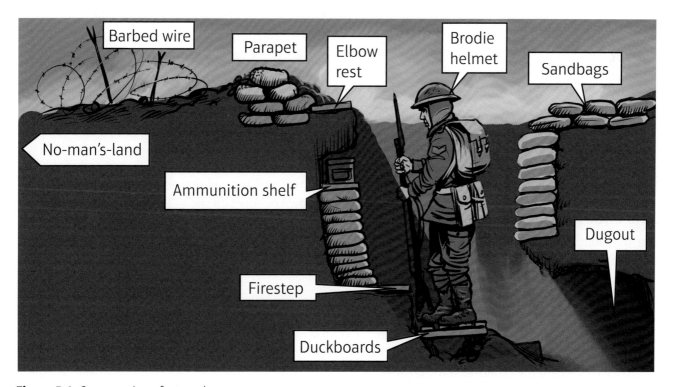

Figure 5.4 Cross section of a trench.

The Ypres Salient*, the Somme, Arras and Cambrai

This section will outline the key battles in the British sector of the Western Front. It will be important to refer back to this section when looking at specific medical advancements on the Western Front.

Key term

Salient*

An area of a battlefield that extends into enemy territory, so that it is surrounded on three sides by the enemy and is therefore in a vulnerable position.

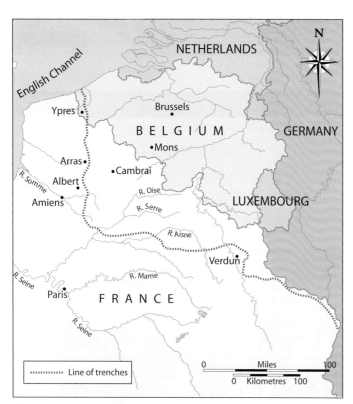

Figure 5.5 Map of the Western Front.

1914: the First Battle of Ypres

During the first months of the war, the BEF had moved to the town of Ypres in western Belgium, in order to prevent the German advance towards the sea. In the autumn of 1914, the Germans launched an attack on the British positions to the east and north-east of Ypres. Although the British lost over 50,000 troops in this battle, which went on from 12 October to 11 November, they held on to Ypres. This meant they controlled the English Channel ports, so that supplies and reinforcements could be provided. By the end of the battle, the Germans had extended their control around the edge of the Ypres Salient as far as the village of Messines.

The use of mines at Hill 60

Hill 60 was a man-made hill to the south-east of Ypres. The Germans had captured it in December 1914 and its height gave them a strategic advantage in this area. The British used the method of offensive mining to take it back in April 1915. This involved tunnelling into and under the hill. Five mines were placed in the tunnels. When they exploded they blew the top off Hill 60 and the British were able to take this strategically important position.

Extend your knowledge

Digging tunnels on the Western Front

The men who joined the Tunnelling Companies had all worked underground before the war – including, for example, coal miners from Northumberland, sewage drain diggers from Manchester and tube tunnel diggers from London. These men were often shorter than the minimum height requirement for the army. They experienced a very high death rate.

1915: the Second Battle of Ypres

As soon as the battle for Hill 60 was finished, the Second Battle of Ypres began. This took place as a sequence of battles over a period of about one month, from 22 April through to 25 May 1915. It is significant in the history of the First World War as it was the first time that the Germans used chlorine gas on the Western Front (see pages 154–155). British losses during this month totalled about 59,000 men. By the end of the battle, the Germans had moved about two miles closer to the town of Ypres on the eastern side of the salient.

1916: the Battle of the Somme

Source C

A still from the 1916 British film, *The Battle of the Somme*.

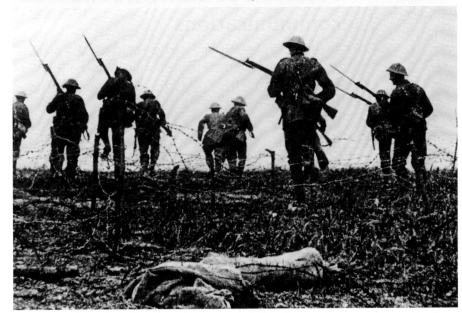

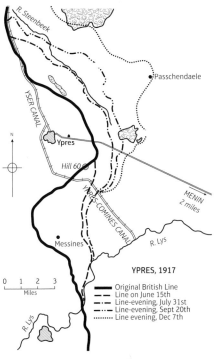

YPRES, 1917

0 1 2 3	—— Original British Line
Miles	– – – Line on June 15th
	–·– Line-evening, July 31st
	–··– Line-evening, Sept 20th
	········ Line evening, Dec 7th

Figure 5.6 Map of the Ypres Salient.

Activity ?

This photograph claimed to show British soldiers advancing at the start of the Battle of the Somme. It is now thought this sequence was staged away from the frontline. Does this affect the way in which you can use the photograph as evidence?

The British attack on the Somme aimed to take ground from the Germans and was launched on 1 July 1916. The casualties on both sides were enormous: on the first day alone, British casualties were over 57,000, with deaths totalling around 20,000 men. The British tried two new strategies, which would both eventually contribute to increased casualty rates:

* **the use of the creeping barrage,** which saw artillery launched from the trenches towards the German lines just ahead of the British infantry as it advanced forwards.
* **the first use of tanks in warfare** – however, the use of tanks had many technical problems and they were not very successful.

By the time the Battle of the Somme ended in November 1916, it is estimated that the British had suffered over 400,000 casualties.

Tunnels, caves and quarries at Arras

The area around Arras is very chalky, and so it is easy to tunnel through. Quarries and tunnels had been dug in this landscape since Roman times. In 1916, the British decided to link the existing tunnels, caves and quarries to create an underground network around Arras to act as shelters against German attacks. They were also built to enable safe underground movement. The work was carried out by Tunnelling Companies from Britain and New Zealand. In total, they dug more than 2.5 miles of tunnels in five months. Up to 25,000 men could be stationed in the tunnels, which contained electric lights, running water, a light railway system and a fully functioning hospital (see page 162).

1917: the Battle of Arras

In April 1917, 24,000 men who had been hiding in tunnels dug near the German trenches attacked. The aim of the offensive was to break through the German lines. In the first few days, it appeared that this aim was achieved, as the British advanced about eight miles. However, as the advance slowed, virtually no further progress was made and by the end of the offensive in May, there was a large number of casualties (nearly 160,000 British and Canadians).

Source D

From 'The General', a poem written by Siegfried Sassoon in 1918. Sassoon served as an officer on the Western Front from 1914. He was treated for shellshock (a psychological condition caused by prolonged exposure to bombardment) in 1917, after which he returned to fight on the Western Front.

"Good morning, good morning," the General said,
When we met him last week on our way to the line.
Now the soldiers he smiled at are most of 'em dead,
And we're cursing his staff for incompetent swine.
"He's a cheery old card," muttered Harry to Jack
As they slogged up to Arras with rifle and pack.
But he did for them both by his plan of attack.

Activities ?

Study Source D.

1   Does the detail in the poem match the events at the Battle of Arras?

2   What questions should you ask before using a poem as a piece of historical evidence?

1917: the Third Battle of Ypres

The purpose of the Third Battle of Ypres in 1917 was for the British army to break out of the Ypres Salient. The British wanted to remove the German advantage of having the higher ground. Throughout June, the British had prepared for the main attack in the battle of Messines, where they had driven the Germans off the ridge that formed part of the Ypres Salient and which the Germans had occupied since October 1914. The British launched their main attack on 31 July, marching east from Ypres towards Passchendaele. The army advanced about two miles on the first day. Soon though, the weather turned to rain and the ground became waterlogged – so much so that many men fell in the mud and drowned. This campaign lasted until November. By then, the British had moved the edge of the salient back by about seven miles. The cost of this advance was an estimated 245,000 British casualties.

1917: the Battle of Cambrai

The Battle of Cambrai was launched on 20 October 1917. The artillery barrage was changed so that less warning of the coming attack was given to the Germans. It was accompanied by the first large-scale use of tanks – nearly five hundred were used in this battle. They were able to move easily across the barbed wire and their machine guns were very effective.

Problems of transport and communications

The constant shelling, and the type of terrain that soldiers were fighting on (similar to the conditions in the Third Battle of Ypres), left the landscape full of craters and holes and destroyed many roads. This led to major problems in transporting injured men away from the frontline. Before the war, this region had been used as farmland, and the use of fertiliser was extensive. This meant there was a lot of bacteria in the soil that could lead to infected wounds.

Men who were injured on the Western Front needed to be moved away from the frontline in stages, as soon as their condition was stable enough. Stretcher bearers, like Edward Munro (see Source E), would carry away the large numbers of wounded from the frontline, both during the day and at night. This meant they often had to expose themselves to shelling and gunfire. Further away from the frontline, it was possible to carry out more advanced medical procedures, and also to provide some protection against shelling. The faster an injury could be treated, the more likely a person was to survive.

Source E

From Edward Munro's *Diaries of a Stretcher Bearer*. This entry comes from 7 November 1916, when Munro was in the Somme.

We commenced to carry down the wounded of whom there were a considerable number. The 7th Brigade had made an attack on the German line the previous night and had suffered many casualties. The country over which we have to carry is most difficult to traverse [walk across], being pitted with shell holes, mostly waterlogged. Fritz [a reference to the Germans] keeps up a fairly constant shelling. Yesterday he caught some of the 6th Ambulance bearers, killing two. In this area was started the system of carrying the stretchers shoulder high — four to a stretcher, this being much less fatiguing than the old method of two carrying with slings... The carrying at night is very trying as there are no clearly defined tracks. The landmarks that serve to guide one in the daytime are not visible at night.

Source F

Stretcher bearers carrying a wounded man to safety at the third battle of Ypres in August 1917. This photograph was taken by Lieutenant John Brooke, an official photographer for the British army on the Western Front.

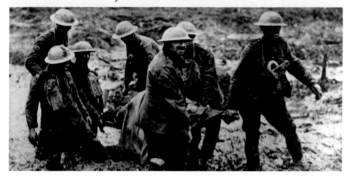

Horse-drawn and motor ambulances

When the BEF was first sent to France in August 1914, the military leadership decided not to send any motor ambulances with them. It was soon realised that this was a mistake, as the horse-drawn ambulance wagons could not cope with the large number of casualties. Men who were transported in these wagons were shaken about, which often made their injuries even worse. This lack of transport actually led to soldiers being left to die or being taken prisoner by the Germans.

When news of this reached Britain, *The Times* newspaper ran a public appeal for donations. By October 1914, after only three weeks, the appeal had raised enough money to buy 512 ambulance wagons, which would make transporting wounded soldiers much easier, and would prevent injuries being made worse from the move. The first motor ambulances were sent to the Western Front in October 1914, as a result of work by the Red Cross. However, motor vehicles could not operate in much of the muddy terrain of the frontline, so horse-drawn

Activities ?

Study Source F.

1 Describe the photo Source F – what is happening?

2 How could a historian use this source for an enquiry into the problems that faced stretcher bearers?

3 What other sources would be helpful in considering the work and problems faced by stretcher bearers on the Western Front?

wagons continued to be used throughout the war. In worse terrain, six horses, rather than the usual two, pulled the ambulance wagons.

Train, barge and ship ambulances

Wounded men might also be transported by train or by canal in the final stage of their evacuation to the Base Hospitals on the French coast (see page 162). In the first few months of the war on the Western Front, the Royal Army Medical Corps (RAMC), which was responsible for medical care in the army (see page 158), had to use French goods trains. The first ambulance train designed for carrying wounded soldiers arrived in France in November 1914. It had spaces for stretchers fitted down both sides of the carriage.

Later, some trains sent to France even contained operating theatres. There were concerns that the numbers of wounded being moved on the railways damaged the war effort because they contributed to too many trains moving around on the rail network of northern France and Belgium. This led to the decision to also make use of canal barges as transport for the wounded to Base Hospitals. Although the journey was slow, it was comfortable, and some of the wounded bypassed the Base Hospitals to be transferred directly onto the ships that were transporting wounded men back to Britain.

Source G

From a speech made by Walter Roch in Parliament, 23 June 1915. Roch was a Liberal MP and was taking part in a debate on how the government should spend its money.

I want to bring to the notice of the House information in connection with the treatment of the wounded in Flanders. The information is not my own personal knowledge, but from several very close personal friends who have been connected with this, although I cannot give their names. I am told that it is of the utmost importance that the men who are wounded should be treated as quickly as possible, and that their wounds should have the best possible attention as soon as may be. The suggestion I have to make is that there should be many more of these evacuation hospitals than there are in France at the present moment, that they should be much better equipped with operating theatres and other appliances, and that they should be more sanitary and hygienic in their nature.

THINKING HISTORICALLY Evidence (1b&c)

The message and the messenger

There are many sources of information about the past. Historians use these sources to help them **draw conclusions**. When information is used to help you form a conclusion, it is used as **evidence**.

Read Source G. In this source, Walter Roch, a Liberal MP, says a number of things. Roch was making a public speech that he knew would be:

a heard in London by his audience

b reported in parliamentary records and possibly in the press

What **information** does the source contain? What was Roch **saying**? Answer the following questions to find out.

1 What does Roch say is important for wounded men?

2 What does he say the conditions in the hospitals should be like?

3 What impression do you think other MPs would have had about Roch's sources of information?

Historians are not usually interested in information for its own sake. Historians are interested in **using** information to work out the **answers** to questions about the past. **Use** the information you have just extracted from the source and the information about its **context** to try and work out answers to the following questions about the way in which Parliament was helping the wounded in 1915.

4 What does Roch's speech suggest about the conditions in hospitals at this date?

5 What do you think Roch wanted Parliament to spend some of its money on?

Summary

- Trench warfare had begun on the Western Front by the end of 1914.
- As the trench system developed, a complex network of trenches was created in which men could live and fight.
- Tunnels and caves at Arras were used as part of the defensive system.
- Chlorine gas was first used by the Germans at the Second Battle of Ypres in 1915.
- The first motorised ambulances sent to France were provided by public donations and organisations such as the British Red Cross.
- Wounded men were moved away from the frontline by trains and canal boats.

Checkpoint

Strengthen

S1 In what ways were the problems of transporting wounded men dealt with?

Challenge

Think about the different types of source used in this section on the context of the British sector of the Western Front.

C1 Using the types of sources from Figure 5.2 (page 142) make a table with one page for each type of source. Divide each page into three columns: 'Example', 'Strengths', 'Weaknesses.'

C2 Fill in this table for Sources A, C and D.

If you are not confident about any of these questions, your teacher can give you some hints.

5.3 Conditions requiring medical treatment on the Western Front

Main medical problems on the Western Front

Conditions in the trenches were very unpleasant. Sanitary, or hygienic, conditions for such large numbers of people posed a problem. In summer, the combination of sewage and dead bodies made the smell dreadful, whilst in winter, bad weather gave rise to both flooding and frostbite. In November and December 1914, there were over 6,000 cases of frostbite. Rat infestation was normal. A number of medical problems were caused by these conditions.

The nature of wounds

Rifles and explosives

In a case study of over 200,000 wounded men admitted to Casualty Clearing Stations (CCS) on the Western Front, it was discovered that high-explosive shells and shrapnel were responsible for 58% of wounds. When a shell exploded, it could kill or injure a soldier immediately. A shell explosion also scattered shrapnel (fragments of metal in the casing), which travelled at fast speeds over a wide area. This meant that anyone who was in the way of the shrapnel was likely to be wounded. About 60% of injuries were to arms and legs.

	Main symptoms	Attempted solutions to deal with the problem
Trench foot	Painful swelling of the feet, caused by standing in cold mud and water. In the second stage of trench foot, gangrene set in. Gangrene is the decomposition of body tissue due to a loss of blood supply.	• Prevention was key. • Rubbing whale oil into feet to protect them. • Keeping feet dry and regularly changing socks. • If gangrene developed, then amputation was the only solution to stop it spreading along the leg.
Trench fever	Flu-like symptoms with high temperature, headache and aching muscles. This condition was a major problem because it affected an estimated half a million men on the Western Front.	• By 1918, the cause of trench fever had been identified as contact with lice. • Delousing stations were set up. After this, there was a decline in the numbers experiencing the condition.
Shellshock	Symptoms included tiredness, headaches, nightmares, loss of speech, uncontrollable shaking and complete mental breakdown. It has been suggested that about 80,000 British troops experienced shellshock.	• The condition was not well understood at the time. • In some cases, such as Siegfried Sassoon and Wilfred Owen, this involved treatment back in Britain. The Craiglockhart Hospital in Edinburgh treated 2,000 men for shellshock. • However, some soldiers who experienced shellshock were accused of cowardice. Many were punished for this – some were even shot.

The case study also found that bullets were responsible for 39% of wounds. Machine guns could fire 450 rounds a minute, and their bullets could fracture bones or pierce organs. Rifles could fire accurately at up to 500 m, but lacked the speed of machine guns.

Shrapnel, wound infection and head injuries

When men were injured, either by shrapnel or by bullets, the metal would penetrate their body, taking with it the fabric of the uniform from the area surrounding the wound. The soil in the region, which had been intensively farmed with large quantities of fertiliser before the war, contained the bacteria for both tetanus and gas gangrene. Gangrene is an infection caused by a lack of blood to an area in the body. Gas gangrene is an infection that produces gas in gangrenous wounds. When wounds were exposed to the soil the presence of these bacteria made infection much more likely. The impact of tetanus was reduced by the use of anti-tetanus injections from the end of 1914. However, there was no cure for gas gangrene. The bacteria for gas gangrene spread though the body quickly and could kill a person within a day.

At the start of the war, the headgear worn by soldiers was a soft cap. To protect against head injuries, a trial using the Brodie helmet was carried out in 1915. This was a steel helmet with a strap that prevented it being thrown off the head in an explosion. It was estimated that it reduced fatal

Source A

From an interview with Captain Maberly Esler in 1974. He was a medical officer. Here he is recalling events at Hooge, in the Ypres salient, in June 1915.

> We'd never attempt any major surgery or anything like that in the trenches — one couldn't do it. The only thing you could do was to cover a wound to keep it from getting infected, or stop a haemorrhage by compression if they were bleeding to death. Several people got tetanus afterwards from an infection in the ground which was carried in shelled areas. The ground had been shelled for such a long time it was in rather a septic sort of condition.

head wounds by 80%, so the helmet was then provided to all soldiers fighting on the Western Front.

The effects of gas attacks

Gas attacks caused great panic and fear, as is shown in Wilfred Owen's poem *Dulce et Decorum Est* in Source B. It was not, however, a major cause of death, with only about 6,000 British soldiers dying as a result of gas attacks. The British army gave troops on the Western Front gas masks from 1915, which became more sophisticated over time. Still, gas attacks were greatly feared by soldiers on the Western Front.

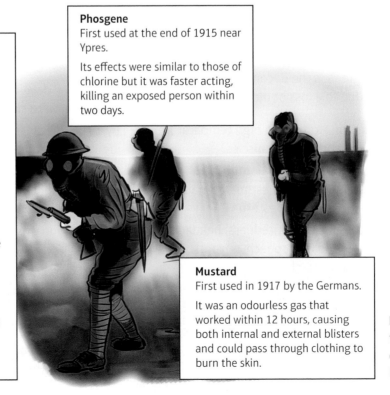

Chlorine
First used by the Germans in 1915 at the second battle of Ypres.

It led to death by suffocation.

The medical services had no experience in dealing with gas attacks, and so had to experiment with treatments.

Gas masks were given to all British troops in July 1915.

Before this, soldiers developed their own system of gas masks. They soaked cotton pads with urine and pressed them to their faces to help stop the gas entering their lungs.

The British retaliated with their own chlorine attack later in 1915 at the Battle of Loos, but the wind changed direction and the gas blew back on the British lines.

Phosgene
First used at the end of 1915 near Ypres.

Its effects were similar to those of chlorine but it was faster acting, killing an exposed person within two days.

Mustard
First used in 1917 by the Germans.

It was an odourless gas that worked within 12 hours, causing both internal and external blisters and could pass through clothing to burn the skin.

Figure 5.7 Three types of gas attacks on the Western Front.

Source B

From '*Dulce et Decorum Est*', a poem written by Wilfred Owen in 1917 whilst he was being treated for shellshock. He served on the Western Front in 1916–17 and returned in 1918, where he was killed in action shortly before the end of the war. The text in the title and the end of the poem is in Latin and means 'it is sweet and fitting to die for one's country'.

```
Gas! Gas! Quick, boys! — An ecstasy of
   fumbling,
Fitting the clumsy helmets just in time;
But someone still was yelling out and
   stumbling,
And flound'ring like a man in fire or lime...
Dim, through the misty panes and thick green
   light,
As under a green sea, I saw him drowning.
In all my dreams, before my helpless sight,
He plunges at me, guttering, choking, drowning.
If in some smothering dreams you too could
   pace
```

```
Behind the wagon that we flung him in,
And watch the white eyes writhing in his face,
His hanging face, like a devil's sick of sin;
If you could hear, at every jolt, the blood
Come gargling from the froth-corrupted lungs,
Obscene as cancer, bitter as the cud
Of vile, incurable sores on innocent tongues,
   —
My friend, you would not tell with such high
   zest
To children ardent for some desperate glory,
The old Lie; Dulce et Decorum est
Pro patria mori.
```

Source C

From the notebook of Lance Sergeant Elmer Cotton, who served in the 5th Northumberland Fusiliers in 1915. He is describing the effects of a chlorine gas attack.

```
It produces a flooding of the lungs. It is
the equivalent to drowning, only on dry
land. The effects are these – a splitting
headache and a terrific thirst (but to drink
water is instant death), a knife-edge pain in
the lungs and the coughing up of a greenish
froth off the stomach and the lungs, finally
resulting in death. It is a fiendish death to
die.
```

Activities ?

1 Study Sources B, C and D.
2 Draw up a table to show the similarities and differences between the three sources when presenting the effects of a gas attack.
3 How much weight do you give to each source separately as a description of the effects of a gas attack?
4 What other sources could you use to find out more about the effects of a gas attack?

Source D

From a 1919 painting by John Singer Sargent. Sargent was commissioned by the British War Memorials Committee to paint this in 1918 and researched the painting by visiting both Arras and Ypres before the end of the war. These soldiers have experienced a mustard gas attack.

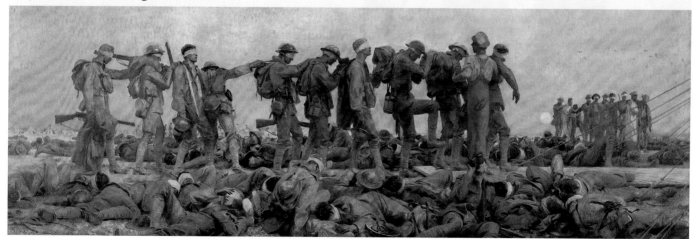

Asking questions: dealing with gas attacks

You need to think about the way sources require historians to ask themselves three sorts of questions. Look at Source E.

Content questions

What can you learn from the content? You can see that the source is a soldier wearing a mask.

Provenance questions

Now you need the caption! How does provenance affect the usefulness of the source? Remember, for provenance, you need to break things down into nature, origin, and purpose.

1 Nature – it is a photograph.
2 Origin comes from the caption – this was taken in the same month that the Second Battle of Ypres began.
3 Purpose can be difficult to determine for a photograph. Might it have been for use as propaganda? In this case, it is hard to think of a propaganda purpose. Does it look like it was set up?

Perhaps it was to inform soldiers about the best way that they could protect themselves against gas attacks.

Context questions

You know two things that are relevant to Source E.

1 The first use of chlorine gas by the Germans took place in April 1915 at the Second Battle of Ypres.
2 The British were not prepared for gas attacks and so they had to experiment to find the best way to protect soldiers.

So, if you were asked how useful Source E is, you could say something like this [key: content, provenance, context]:

'Source E is useful because it shows the first attempts to make a gas mask. Although we don't know why the photo was taken, it might have been set up so that soldiers could learn how best to protect themselves. We know that proper gas masks were not provided at the time because the gas attacks were unexpected.'

What this does (and what you can do) is explain why the source is useful, using criteria you have explained based on the three types of question.

Source E

Photograph of a man wearing a cotton wool pad respirator, April 1915. This was a simple form of gas mask. The Second Battle of Ypres also began in April 1915.

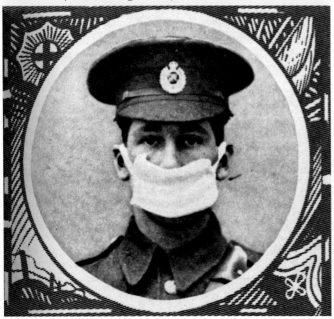

Source F

From the autobiography of Geoffrey Keynes, *The Gates of Memory* (1981). This account was originally published in 1968. Keynes was important in developing blood transfusions during the war.

On 6 February 1915 I was detailed for duty on an ambulance train. The numbers of patients carried on each journey varied between 100 and 400. During my turn of duty in the train we carried nearly 19,000 patients. Medical duties were usually restricted to ensuring that the wounded men, who had already been attended in a Dressing Station or Casualty Clearing Station travelled as comfortably as possible with the help of sedative and pain-killing drugs. Frequently they had to suffer violent jolts during shunting operations.

Usually the patients had been fully cared for before being sent on by train to the base hospitals, but on one occasion (12 March 1915), the train was ordered to go close to the frontline and take on casualties who had barely received first aid.

Now look at Sources F and G. The content of Source F describes the work done by doctors on an ambulance train. Although the provenance tells us that this was written many years later, the detailed references to dates and figures in the source suggests that the writer kept a diary and that he is using this to help him remember what happened. Source G, on the other hand, is clearly a historical photograph, preserving a moment in time. We don't know exactly what date this photograph was taken – only the month and year. Its purpose was to record the awful conditions that faced men on the Western Front. Both sources tell you something about the different types of transport that were used to carry the wounded to safety and treatment.

Source G

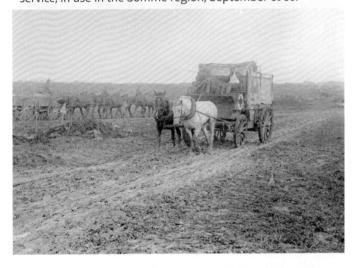

A photograph of a wagon belonging to the Field Ambulance service, in use in the Somme region, September 1916.

Activities

1 Explain the differences between questions for comprehension, questions for context, and prompted questions.

2 Pick a source that could be used by a historian who was studying day-to-day life in your school now.

   a Describe the source.

   b Give an example of a comprehension question that could be asked about the source, and explain what you would learn from it.

   c Give an example of a provenance question (nature, origin, purpose) that could be asked about the source and explain what you would learn from it.

   d Give an example of a context question that could be asked about the source, and explain what you would learn from it.

3 Give an example of a question or enquiry prompted by the source, and explain why this would be an interesting enquiry to follow.

Summary

- Common medical problems that faced men fighting on the Western Front faced were trench foot, trench fever and shellshock.
- The introduction of the Brodie helmet saved many lives by protecting the head against shrapnel injuries.
- Gas attacks caused burning skin and suffocation.

Checkpoint

Strengthen

S1 Explain all the medical problems and possible injuries that soldiers faced in the trenches that are referred to in this section. Then note down all the solutions to the problems.

Challenge

C1 How useful are Sources B, C and D on the effects of gas attacks on the Western Front?

If you are not confident about any of these questions, form a group with other students, discuss the answers and then record your conclusions. Your teacher can give you some hints.

5.4 The work of the RAMC and FANY

Learning outcomes

- Understand the main stages of the chain of evacuation and what happened to wounded soldiers at each stage.
- Know about the role played by the RAMC* and FANY* in dealing with wounded soldiers.

Key terms

RAMC*

Royal Army Medical Corps. This branch of the army was responsible for medical care and was formally founded in 1898.

FANY*

First Aid Nursing Yeomanry. Founded in 1907, this was the first women's voluntary organisation to send volunteers to the Western Front. It provided frontline support for the medical services, for example by driving ambulances and engaging in emergency first aid.

Source A

From F. S. Brereton, *The Great War and the RAMC*, published in 1919. Brereton served as a Lieutenant-Colonel in the RAMC on the Western Front. This is a diagram showing how the chain of evacuation might operate in theory.

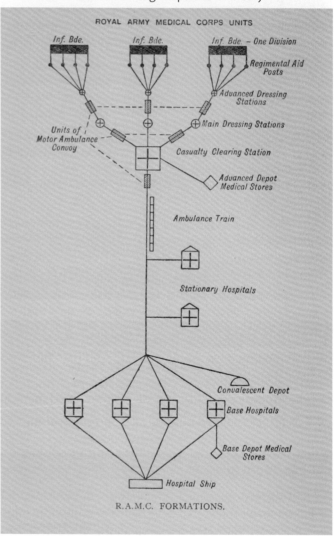

R.A.M.C. FORMATIONS.

To deal with the large numbers of casualties in the First World War, the number of medical professionals needed to be increased dramatically.

The table below shows the number of medical professionals in 1914 and 1918.

	1914	1918
Medical officers	3,168	13,063
Other ranks (e.g. private)	16,331	131,099

More than half of Britain's doctors were serving with the armed forces and most of these were deployed to the Western Front.

The system of transport and the stages of treatment

Because of the large numbers of casualties, it was essential that there was an efficient system to get the wounded from the frontline to a safe area where they could be treated. This system became known as the **chain of evacuation.**

The main stages in the chain of evacuation were **Regimental Aid Posts (RAP), Dressing Stations (ADS and MDS), Casualty Clearing Stations** and **Base Hospitals**. Remember – these were the main stages, but were not always followed in the same order for every casualty.

158

Source B

From Ward Muir's *Observations of an Orderly*, published in 1917. Muir was a Lance Corporal in the RAMC and worked in a hospital in London that received patients from the Western Front at the end of the chain of evacuation.

We orderlies meet each convoy at the front door of the hospital. The walking-cases are the first to arrive — men who are either not ill enough, or not badly enough wounded, to need to be put on stretchers in ambulances. They come from the station in motor-cars supplied by the London Ambulance Column. The few minutes which the walking-case spends in the receiving hall are occupied in drinking a cup of cocoa, and in 'having his particulars taken'. Poor soul! — he is weary of giving his 'particulars'. He has had to give them half-a-dozen times at least, perhaps more, since he left the front. At the field dressing-station they wanted his particulars, at the clearing-station, on the train, at the base hospital, on another train, on the steamer, on the next train, and now in this English hospital.

Activities ?

Study Source A and Source B. When Source B refers to 'particulars' it means personal details.

1 Why do you think the first thing that happened to the new arrivals was that they were given a cup of cocoa and had their 'particulars' taken?

2 How useful are these two sources in helping to establish the key stages in the chain of evacuation?

3 What other sources would give you useful information on the chain of evacuation? Think of as many as possible. Now compare your list with a partner. Decide which would be the most useful.

Regimental Aid Post (RAP)

The RAP was generally located within 200 m of the frontline, in communication trenches or deserted buildings. It was made up of a Regimental Medical Officer, with some help from stretcher bearers with first-aid knowledge. Wounded men would either walk in themselves or be carried in by other soldiers. The purpose of the RAP was to give immediate first aid and to get as many men back to the fighting as possible. It could not deal with serious injuries. These had to be moved to the next stage in the chain of evacuation.

Dressing Stations (ADS and MDS)

In theory, there should have been an Advanced Dressing Station (ADS) about 400 m from the RAP and a Main Dressing Station (MDS) a further half a mile back. In practice, this was often not the case – and there may only have been one Dressing Station. Where possible, the Dressing Stations were located in abandoned buildings, dug-outs or bunkers, in order to offer protection from enemy shelling. Where these were not available, tents would be used. Each dressing station would be staffed by ten medical officers, plus medical orderlies and stretcher bearers of the RAMC. From 1915, there were also some nurses available for this part of the chain of evacuation. To get to the Dressing Station, men would either walk, if they were able to do so, or be carried in by stretcher in stages.

Source C

From the diary of E.S.B. Hamilton, 19 August 1916. Hamilton had been in France for over a year at this time, as part of the Field Ambulance. At the time of this diary entry, he was working at an Advanced Dressing Station on the Somme.

The dugout [of the ADS] is awfully overcrowded both night and day and it is impossible to get it cleaned or aired. [There were] something like 800 people through here in about thirty hours the day before yesterday. This is far too much work for the personnel [of] three officers and about 115 men. Result [is] a lot of the men are done up and the officers seedy and depressed.

Extend your knowledge

John McCrae

John McCrae was a Canadian medical offer serving on the Western Front. He treated many wounded soldiers during the Second Battle of Ypres. The famous war poem *In Flanders Fields*, written by McCrae, was composed at the Essex Farm Advanced Dressing Station in May, 1915. The remains of this dressing station can still be seen today.

Source D

A photograph of an Advanced Dressing Station. This was taken in August 1916 at Pozieres Ridge, which was part of the Somme campaign.

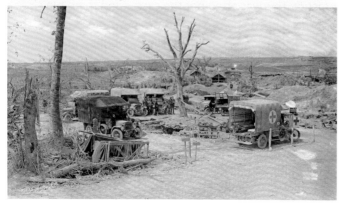

Those working at the Dressing Stations belonged to a unit of the RAMC called the **Field Ambulance**. This should not be confused with the vehicles that carried the sick and wounded, which were known as **ambulance wagons**. In theory, each Field Ambulance unit could deal with 150 wounded men, but when major battles were taking place, they would have to deal with many more. The Field Ambulance at Hooge in the Ypres Salient dealt with about 1,000 casualties on 10–11 August 1917. The Field Ambulance units did not have the facilities to tend to wounded men for more than a week. Men who had been treated would either be returned to their units if they were fit enough to fight again, or they would be moved on to the next phase of the chain of evacuation by horse or motor ambulance.

Casualty Clearing Stations (CCS)

Casualty Clearing Stations were located a sufficient distance from the frontline to provide some safety against attack, but close enough to be accessible by ambulance wagons. Often the CCS closest to the frontline would specialise in operating on the most critical injuries, such as those to the chest. They were set up in buildings such as factories or schools and were often located near to a railway line to allow the next stage of the chain of evacuation to take place quickly.

When wounded soldiers arrived here, they were divided into three groups. This system was called **triage**, from the French word for sorting or selecting. Triage helped medical staff make decisions about treatment.

The three categories the wounded were divided into are:

1 **The walking wounded**. These were the men who could be patched up and returned to the fighting.

2 **Those in need of hospital treatment**. These men would need to be transported to a Base Hospital once they had been treated for any immediate life-threatening injuries.

3 **Those who were so severely wounded that there was no chance of recovery**. These men would be made comfortable, but the medical resources available were given to those who were more likely to survive their wounds.

Here are some useful statistics about the CCS during the Third Battle of Ypres in 1917.

- There were 24 CCS in the Ypres Salient.
- 379 doctors and 502 nurses treated more than 200,000 casualties.
- The medical staff operated on 30% of the men who were admitted.
- In total, 3.7% of the men admitted died.

Exam-style question, Section A

How useful are Sources C and D for an enquiry into the treatment of the wounded at ADSs on the Western Front?

Explain your answer, using Sources C and D and your knowledge of the historical context. **8 marks**

Exam tip

Go through these steps when preparing your answer.

- Always concentrate on the enquiry – in this question, the treatment of the wounded at ADSs, and then identify points from the content.
- Think about the provenance (nature, origin, purpose) of both sources.
- Think about what you know about the context – the Advanced Dressing Stations.
- Link together the content, provenance and context in your answer and include how the provenance and context affects the usefulness of the content.

Source E

Photograph of a ward in the Casualty Clearing Station at Hazebrouck in 1915. Hazebrouck was close to Ypres.

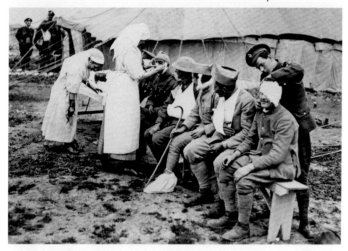

Activities ?

In pairs, study the statistics about the Casualty Clearing Stations during the Third Battle of Ypres and Source E.

1 What do you learn from the statistics?

2 Why can statistics be useful to historians?

3 What problems should historians be aware of when using statistics?

4 Describe the main features of the Casualty Clearing Station in the photograph.

5 What evidence does Source E provide that medical treatment in the Casualty Clearing Stations was effective?

The role of FANY

The first six FANYs arrived in France on 27 October 1914. However, the British would not make use of them so they devoted their energies to helping French and Belgian troops.

Finally, in January 1916, the British army decided to allow FANYs to drive ambulances. They became the first women to carry out this role, replacing British Red Cross male ambulance drivers. They were used to transport wounded troops by ambulance in the Calais region. Although there were never more than 450 FANYs in France, they did open the way for other women who were attached to other organisations, such as the Voluntary Aid Detachments (VADs), to participate in the frontline.

Extend your knowledge

What else did FANY do?

FANY did things other than driving ambulances to support the soldiers on the Western Front.

- They drove supplies such as food and clothes to the frontline.
- They had a mobile bath unit which provided baths to the soldiers in water heated by the power from the van's engine.
- They set up cinemas to help the morale of soldiers.

Source F

From Pat Beauchamp's autobiography, *Fanny Goes to War*, published in 1919. Beauchamp first worked as a nurse, bringing in the wounded from the trenches, and from 1916 as an ambulance driver. Here she is writing about an account of FANYs from an English newspaper.

The following is an extract from an account by Mr. Beach Thomas in a leading daily: "Our Yeomanry nurses who, among other work, drive, clean, and manage their own ambulance cars… have done prodigies [wonders] along the Belgian front. One of their latest activities has been to devise and work a peripatetic [travelling] bath… Ten collapsible baths are packed into a motor car which circulates behind the lines. The water is heated by the engine in a cistern in the interior of the car and offers the luxury of a hot bath to several score men."

Base Hospitals

Base Hospitals on the Western Front were located near the French and Belgian coast, so that the wounded men who were treated there would be close to the ports, from which they could be transported home to Britain. At the start of the war there were two types of Base Hospital – the Stationary Hospital and the General Hospital. However, in practice, they worked in very similar ways. Men were treated in both types of hospital until they could be returned to Britain for further treatment or were fit enough to return to the fighting.

As the war progressed, Casualty Clearing Stations played an increasingly important role in dealing with wounds, instead of Base Hospitals. It had become clear that if contaminated wounds were not dealt with quickly, wounded men were more likely to develop gangrene. This meant that the CCSs started doing operations that it was originally believed would be done in the Base Hospitals.

By May 1916, for example, at Number 26 General Hospital at Étaples, most head and chest patients had been operated upon before their arrival at the Base Hospital there. In turn, the Base Hospitals became increasingly responsible for continuing treatment that was begun in the CCSs, before men were either returned to frontline fighting or transported back to Britain. The size of the Base Hospitals increased, especially after a major offensive had taken place. In 1917, three new Base Hospitals with a total of 2,500 beds were available.

As the Base Hospitals were not carrying out their intended role, other important roles emerged for them. They experimented with new techniques which, once successful, were used in the CCSs. For example, by dividing patients up into different wards according to their wounds, such as amputees, head wounds, chest wounds, and by allocating doctors to a specialised ward, it was possible for doctors to become expert in the treatment of particular wounds.

The Casualty Clearing Stations retained their role as the most important place for operations until the spring of 1918. The static nature of trench warfare had meant that the CCSs had been relatively safe early on in the war, but in March 1918, the Germans launched the Spring Offensive. This was a last-ditch attempt to win the war before American troops arrived in Europe and joined the British. It resulted in many CCSs having to move back, so much of the surgery that was required for the wounded was now undertaken again in the Base Hospitals.

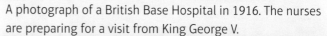
Extend your knowledge

'Blighty' wounds

A 'Blighty' wound, was a wound serious enough to get soldiers away from the fighting and back to Britain via the chain of evacuation, but would not result in permanent medical problems.

Source G

A photograph of a British Base Hospital in 1916. The nurses are preparing for a visit from King George V.

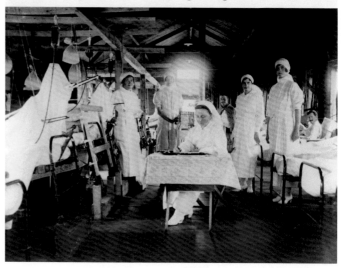

The underground hospital at Arras

In November 1916, tunnelling began under the town of Arras. In 800 m of tunnels, a fully working hospital was created so close to the frontline that it was, in reality, a Dressing Station. From here, wounded soldiers would move through the chain of evacuation. It was sometimes called **Thompson's Cave** after the RAMC officer who was responsible for equipping it. There were waiting rooms for the wounded, 700 spaces where stretchers could be placed as beds, an operating theatre, rest stations for stretcher bearers, and a mortuary to lay out the dead. Electricity and piped water were supplied to the hospital. The hospital was abandoned during the Battle of Arras in 1917, when it was hit by a shell which destroyed the water supply, but luckily did not injure any people.

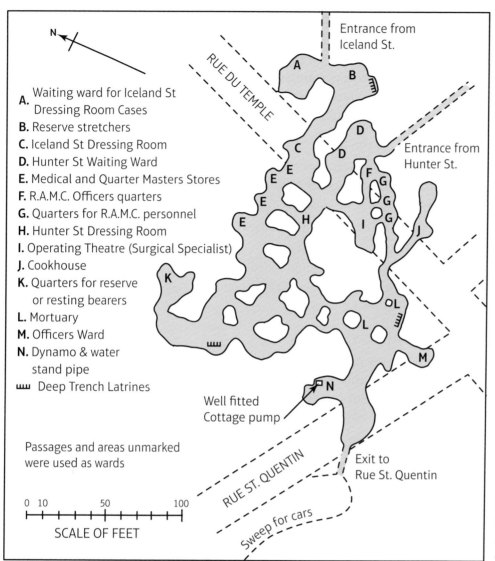

A. Waiting ward for Iceland St Dressing Room Cases
B. Reserve stretchers
C. Iceland St Dressing Room
D. Hunter St Waiting Ward
E. Medical and Quarter Masters Stores
F. R.A.M.C. Officers quarters
G. Quarters for R.A.M.C. personnel
H. Hunter St Dressing Room
I. Operating Theatre (Surgical Specialist)
J. Cookhouse
K. Quarters for reserve or resting bearers
L. Mortuary
M. Officers Ward
N. Dynamo & water stand pipe
⊔⊔⊔ Deep Trench Latrines

Passages and areas unmarked were used as wards

0 10   50   100
SCALE OF FEET

Figure 5.8 Plan of the Arras Underground hospital, also known as Thompson's Cave, based on a drawing from April 1917.

Source H

From Major-General Sir W. G. Macpherson, *Medical Services General History*, published in 1924. Macpherson was on the Western Front from 1914. From 1916–18, he was in charge of the RAMC. He wrote this history based on official records to which he had access. Here he is writing about the underground hospital at Arras.

Dressing Stations were established in caves, cellars and basements of buildings, protected as strongly as possible with sandbags on the outskirts of the town. The chief of these was in a large subterranean cave, from which stone had been excavated for building the town in the 16th century. It was close to the 3rd Division trenches and only 800 yards from the frontline. Two entrances for stretchers were tunnelled into it from the communication trenches, and an exit tunnelled out from the back into Rue St Quentin, where an approach was constructed for ambulance cars. This cave was fitted with electric light and a piped water supply and was able to accommodate 700 wounded on stretchers in two tiers.

Source I

From *The Daily Telegraph*, a British newspaper, 29 April 1915.

POISON BOMBS: CANADIAN'S HEROIC CONDUCT

There appears little doubt that the material used by the Germans in the "poison bombs" is chlorine. This is the only conclusion one can arrive at after hearing the graphic narration of a Canadian who was enveloped in the fumes near Ypres.

The Canadian said, "Directly we opened fire the Germans rained shrapnel over us. We kept the guns going, wounded as some of us were. That we could stand. We had no complaints, because it was honest warfare. Then came the surprise. We saw bombs burst in the air and throw off a greenish-yellow vapour..."

At yesterday's meeting of the London Education Committee, the chairman (Mr. Gilbert) called attention to the request of the Government for respirators [gas masks] for the troops.

Using the range of sources

Following up an enquiry

In the examination, you are asked to suggest a possible question and a type of source that you could use to follow up another source. The framework of the question helps you through the four-stage process.

1 The detail you might follow up is the request for respirators.

2 The question you might ask is 'How many gas masks were given to Canadian troops after April 1915?'

3 There are lots of different types of source in this unit. You could suggest private diaries, local newspapers or official records.

4 Lastly, you have to explain the reason for your choice. For example, you could say that you would follow up Source I with a private diary because because gas attacks would be a common event soliders would write about in their diaries.

National newspapers

Source I shows you some of the strengths and weaknesses of national newspapers as sources. The report refers to events that are going on in both the Western Front and at home in response to these events. The chairman of the London Education Committee is named, but the soldier is anonymous. He is only referred to as 'the Canadian'. The article appears to give valid information, but it is also a form of propaganda.

Activities ?

Read Source I in small groups.

a What can you find about the German attack at Ypres, the types of weapon used and the response at home?

b Which of the things you discovered would you also expect to find in a local newspaper?

c How useful is this national newspaper for studying gas attacks?

Summary

- The Royal Army Medical Corps (RAMC) provided both doctors and other staff to support the medical services.
- The First Aid Nursing Yeomanry (FANY) provided additional support to the RAMC.
- Moving the wounded from the frontline to the appropriate medical facility was known as the chain of evacuation.
- The main stages for the most severely wounded were the Regimental Aid Post, the Dressing Station, Casualty Clearing Station and Base Hospitals.

Checkpoint

Strengthen

S1 Create a flow diagram that shows the main stages in the chain of evacuation.

Challenge

C1 How useful are Sources C on page 149 and I on page 164 for a study of government use of propaganda?

If you are not sure, go back to the text in this section to find the details you need.

5.5 The significance of the Western Front for experiments in surgery and medicine

Learning outcomes

- Understand how the experience of war on the Western Front gave rise to new techniques in medical treatment.
- Understand how new methods of surgery developed to treat the large number of head injuries that were a result of trench warfare.

New techniques in the treatment of wounds and infection

A major problem that faced the RAMC at the start of the war on the Western Front was dealing with infections caused by gas gangrene. It was not possible to perform aseptic surgery in Dressing Stations and Casualty Clearing Stations, due to the contaminated conditions and because of the large numbers of wounded men needing treatment.

Because of this, other methods of treatment had to be found. This led to much disagreement in the medical profession between those medics who were facing the frontline conditions on a daily basis, and those who were back in Britain, unfamiliar with what medics in the trenches were facing.

Extend your knowledge

Amputations

Queen Mary's Hospital at Roehampton, just outside London, became the leading centre for fitting new limbs for men who had experienced amputations. Opening in 1915, it had fitted artificial limbs to more than 26,000 men by the end of the war in 1918.

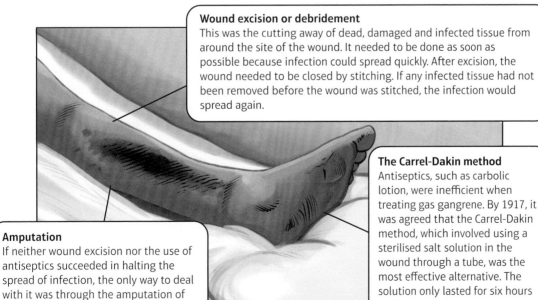

Wound excision or debridement
This was the cutting away of dead, damaged and infected tissue from around the site of the wound. It needed to be done as soon as possible because infection could spread quickly. After excision, the wound needed to be closed by stitching. If any infected tissue had not been removed before the wound was stitched, the infection would spread again.

The Carrel-Dakin method
Antiseptics, such as carbolic lotion, were inefficient when treating gas gangrene. By 1917, it was agreed that the Carrel-Dakin method, which involved using a sterilised salt solution in the wound through a tube, was the most effective alternative. The solution only lasted for six hours and so had to be made as it was needed. This could be difficult, especially when large numbers of wounded men needed treatment at the same time.

Amputation
If neither wound excision nor the use of antiseptics succeeded in halting the spread of infection, the only way to deal with it was through the amputation of wounded limbs. By 1918, 240,000 men had lost limbs – many of them because it was the only way to prevent the spread of infection and death.

Figure 5.9 The main techniques used to prevent infections from spreading.

Source A

From the diary of B. C. Jones, 1915–16. Jones served with the Royal Field Artillery in France from the start of the war until he was wounded in 1915.

7 December. A German shell hit the dugout of our telephone pit. I remembered no more until I woke up in Bethune Casualty Clearing Station Number 33, where I find I have been severely wounded. Left hand blown off, left arm ripped up 12 inches. Scalp wound 6 inches, wound on over side of knee (left) 5 inches.

9 December. Operation on upper arm for gangrene (successful).

12 December. I remain here for 8 days then removed to St Omer by hospital barge, very comfortable. I am then removed by train to Étaples. I am sent to England on the Hospital Ship. Return to Nottingham where I am in bed until the end of February.

3 June 1916. I am eventually transferred to Brighton where I am operated on and re-amputated. Awaiting Roehampton for artificial limb.

Source B

From Ward Muir's Observations of an Orderly, published in 1917. Muir was a Lance Corporal in the RAMC and worked in a hospital in London that received patients from the Western Front at the end of the chain of evacuation.

The majority of stretcher-cases... reach us in a by no means desperate state, for, as I say, they seldom come to England without having been treated previously at a base abroad (except during the periods of heavy fighting). And it is remarkable how often the patient refuses help in getting off the stretcher on to the bed. He may be a cocoon of bandages, but he will courageously heave himself overboard, from stretcher to bed, with a wallop which would be deemed rash even in a person in perfect health.

Activities ?

Study Sources A and B.

1 What conclusions can you draw from the fact that the soldier in Source A needed to have a limb re-amputated when he returned to England?

2 With a partner, make a list of inquiries you think Source A and B would be useful for.

The Thomas splint

In 1914 and 1915, men with a gunshot or shrapnel wound to the leg only had a 20% chance of survival. This was because these wounds created a compound fracture where the broken bone pierced the skin. It was particularly serious if the femur (thigh bone) was fractured, because a large amount of muscle would be damaged. This meant there was likely to be major bleeding into the thigh.

The splint that was in use as the wounded man was transferred from the frontline did not keep the leg rigid. By the time the wounded man arrived at the Casualty Clearing Station, where he could be operated on, he would have lost a great deal of blood, was likely to be in shock and might already have developed gas gangrene in the wound. This combination of factors reduced his chances of surviving an operation to the wound. Many of those who survived did so because their wounded leg was amputated.

It was clear that a way of improving the survival rate for men with this type of injury was needed. In fact, the solution, which only came into use in 1916, had been available since well before the start of the war.

In the late 19th century, Robert Jones worked with his uncle, Hugh Thomas, in his medical practice, where his uncle had designed a splint to stop joints from moving. When the war broke out, Jones was 57 years old. He offered his services immediately to the war effort. He worked with disabled soldiers in a hospital in London and started to make use of his uncle's **Thomas splint**.

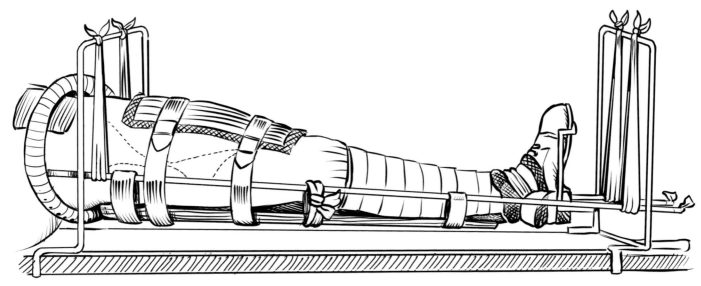

Figure 5.10 The Thomas splint.

As a result of this, in December 1915, he was sent to Boulogne to instruct medical practitioners on how to use the Thomas splint. The introduction of its use from this time increased the survival rate for this type of wound from 20% to 82%.

The use of mobile x-ray units

Extend your knowledge

Marie Curie

Marie Curie was a leading Polish-French scientist who did ground-breaking work on radioactivity. When the war broke out, she immediately understood the importance of x-rays for detecting shrapnel and was responsible for equipping 20 mobile x-ray vans to work in the French sector of the Western Front. These vans were known as 'petites Curies' – little Curies.

X-rays were used from the start of the war. Their main use was to identify shell fragments and bullets in wounds, which, if not removed when the person was wounded, could cause infection. Two x-rays would be taken from different angles and this helped the surgeon to identify quite accurately the location of shrapnel and bullets in the body.

Although a relative success, there were some problems with the use of x-rays for medical practitioners on the Western Front.

- X-rays could not detect all objects in the body. For example, fragments of clothing that were driven into wounds with shrapnel would not show up on an x-ray. However, doctors soon realised that they needed to look for these fragments in the same area as shrapnel when operating on the wounded.

- The length of time that a wounded man had to remain still whilst the x-ray was taken was still several minutes, which could cause problems depending on the wound.

- The tubes used in x-ray machines were fragile and overheated quite quickly. This meant that x-ray machines could only be used for about one hour at a time and then had to be left to cool down. This posed a problem when there was a major offensive going on and large numbers of wounded men were being brought in. The solution was to have three machines which would be used in rotation. When a machine became too hot to continue working, it would be replaced by another one. There had been an advance made in the technology of tubes in the USA by William Coolidge in 1913, but this was not available to the RAMC on the Western Front until the USA entered the war in 1917.

Source C

From *Radiography and Radiotherapeutics*, by Robert Knox, published in 1917. This was a textbook on the use of x-rays written by a British doctor.

```
The need for portable
outfits in connection with
the war has led to a great
development in the provision
of motor wagons containing
complete x-ray apparatus
with all accessories. The
mechanism used for driving
the wagon i.e. the motor
is coupled with a powerful
dynamo which delivers a
continuous current.
```

Exam-style question, Section A

How could you follow up Source C to find out more about x-rays on the Western Front?

In your answer, you must give the question you would ask and the type of source you could use.

Copy out and complete the table below. **4 marks**

Detail in Source C that I would follow up	
Question I would ask	
What type of source I could use	
How this might help answer my question	

Exam tip

This question involves a four-stage process. The example shows you what to do at each stage.

- **Pick a detail.** For example, 'a great development in the provision of motor wagons.'
- **Question I would ask.** How many x-ray vehicles were used in 1917 on the Western Front?
- **Type of source I would use.** Military records showing the number of x-ray vehicles being used in 1917 on the Western Front.
- **How this might help answer my question.** The data would show whether the numbers increased and quantify the words 'great development' in the statement in Source C..

Source D

A photograph of a mobile x-ray unit, taken in 1917. Notice how the equipment has been laid out.

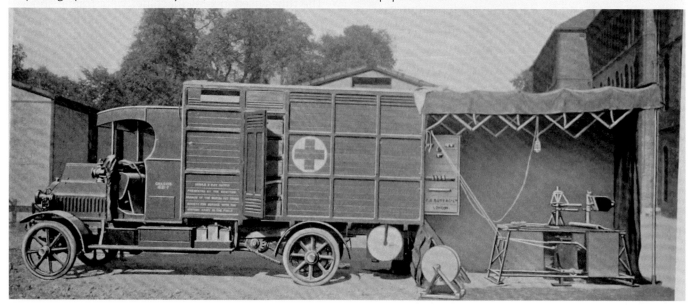

The Base Hospitals and some of the larger Casualty Clearing Stations had static (unmoving) x-ray machines as part of their equipment. Those that did not have them could call on a mobile unit. There were six mobile x-ray units operating in the British sector on the Western Front. Setting up the equipment from the mobile unit took some time. A tent was attached to the back of the van with a table where stretchers could be placed. The x-ray machine was set up next to this table and linked to the engine of the van, which was used to power the x-ray machine. The equipment for processing the x-ray films was set up inside the van. Although the quality of the x-rays taken by the mobile units was not quite as good as that taken by static units, it was sufficient to identify shrapnel and bullets and prevent infection for many of the wounded soldiers (see Source D).

Blood transfusions

The use of blood transfusions from 1915 in the British sector of the Western Front was pioneered by a Canadian doctor, Lawrence Bruce Robertson, in the Base Hospital at Boulogne. He used the indirect method, where a syringe and tube was used to transfer the donor blood to the patient. The purpose of this was to stop the patient going into shock through blood loss before surgery. Even where a wound was relatively minor, shock could kill a soldier. Those who did not experience a negative reaction to the blood transfusion generally recovered. As blood transfusions proved so successful at the Base Hospital, it was decided to extend their use. Therefore, by 1917, blood transfusions were being administered in the Casualty Clearing Stations as a routine measure in the treatment of shock.

Geoffrey Keynes, a British doctor and lieutenant in the RAMC, designed a portable blood transfusion kit that was used to provide blood transfusions close to the frontline. Despite Robertson's pioneering work, this kit did not use stored blood because of the difficulties in keeping the blood fresh when there was no refrigeration available. Keynes added a device to the blood bottle to regulate the flow of the blood which helped prevent clotting. In 1915, Keynes used the new method in a Casually Clearing Station on the Western Front. By his own accounts, it saved countless lives.

The blood bank at Cambrai

The identification of blood groups and the use of blood type O as a universal donor blood type meant that the risk of being transfused with the wrong blood group was reduced (see page 144). The problem of clotting remained, and there was never enough blood on hand to meet demand. However, as the war continued, some advances were made in the storage of blood.

- In 1915, American doctor Richard Lewisohn discovered that by adding sodium citrate to blood, the need for donor-to-donor transfusion was removed. Blood transfusions could be done indirectly, with patients not needing to be in the same room.
- In the same year, Richard Weil discovered that blood with sodium citrate could be refrigerated and stored for up to two days.
- In 1916, Francis Rous and James Turner found that by adding a citrate glucose solution to blood, it could be stored for a much longer period – up to four weeks.

The use of stored blood was clearly demonstrated in 1917 at the Battle of Cambrai. Before the battle, Oswald Hope Robertson, a British-born American doctor, stored 22 units of universal donor blood in glass bottles. He built a carrying case for the bottles in ammunition boxes which he packed with ice and sawdust. He called this a 'blood depot'. During the battle, he treated 20 severely wounded Canadian soldiers with the 22 units of blood, some of which had been collected 26 days before use. They were so badly affected by shock that none of them were expected to survive. In fact, of the 20 wounded men, 11 survived.

Robertson's work at Cambrai was the first time stored blood was used to treat soldiers in shock, and, although it was only on a small scale, demonstrated its potential to save lives. This was important, because during times of heavy fighting, only the most severely wounded were taken to the Casualty Clearing Stations. The less severely wounded, who were normally the men who gave blood for transfusions, would not be taken there. Therefore, the availability of blood stored in a number of blood depots made a huge difference to men's chances of survival.

The attempts to deal with increased numbers of head injuries

About 20% of all wounds in the British sector of the Western Front were to the head, face and neck. This was the part of the body that was most exposed in the trench warfare of the Western Front. Injuries of this nature could be caused by both bullets and shrapnel.

Brain Surgery

Injuries to the brain were very likely to prove fatal at the start of the war because:

- the issue of infection applied just as much to head injuries as it did to wounds to other parts of the body
- there were difficulties involved in moving men with head injuries through the chain of evacuation, as they were often unconscious or confused
- there were very few doctors who had experience of neurosurgery* before the war.

Key term

Neurosurgery*

Surgery carried out on the nervous system, especially the brain and the spine.

Despite the inexperience of doctors in dealing with head wounds, observation quickly led to improvements in methods of treatment.

Harvey Cushing, an American neurosurgeon, developed new techniques in brain surgery on the Western Front. He experimented, for example, with the use of a magnet to remove metal fragments from the brain. He also used a local anaesthetic* rather than a general anaesthetic* when operating. The reason for this was that the brain swelled as a result of general anaesthetics and this increased the risks of the operation. His methods

Observation	New method of treatment
Men who were operated on quickly were more likely to survive.	Specific Casualty Clearing Stations became chosen as centres for brain surgery. For example, during the Third Battle of Ypres, all head injuries were moved to the Casualty Clearing Station at Mendinghem.
It was dangerous to move men too soon after an operation.	Patients remained at the Casualty Clearing Station for three weeks after surgery.
Injuries that looked fairly minor could be hiding more severe injuries.	All head wounds were always carefully examined.

became more effective as he learned more through observation. He operated on 45 patients in 1917 with an operation survival rate of 71%, compared to the general survival rate of 50% for brain surgery.

Key terms

Local anaesthetic*

Keeping a patient awake during an operation, with the area being operated on numbed to prevent pain.

General anaesthetic*

Putting a patient to sleep during an operation.

Source E

From *A Surgeon's Journal 1915–18*, by Harvey Cushing, published in 1936. Here he is describing the conditions under which he is working during the battle of Passchendaele on 19 August 1917.

```
My prize patient, Baker, with the shrapnel
ball removed from his brain, after doing well
for three days suddenly shot up a temperature
to 104 last night about midnight. I took
him to the operating theatre, reopened the
perfectly healed external wound, and found
to my dismay a massive gas infection of
the brain. I bribed two orderlies to stay
up with him in the operating room, where
he could have constant thorough irrigation
over the brain and through the track of
the missile [passing a warm saline solution
along the path taken by the shrapnel to
prevent infection]. No light except candles
was permitted last night.
```

Plastic Surgery

The development of plastic surgery was largely the work of a New Zealand doctor called Harold Gillies. In civilian life, he was an ENT (ear, nose and throat) surgeon. He was sent to the Western Front in January 1915. There he met Charles Valadier, a French man who had been working for the British Red Cross as a dentist since October 1914. Head injuries that might not kill, could cause severe disfigurement. This led Gillies to become interested in facial reconstruction – how to replace and restore those parts of the face that had been destroyed. As he had no background in this type of surgery, he devised new operations to deal with problems as they confronted him.

Activities ?

Study Source E and answer the following questions:

1 Why do you think Baker was Cushing's 'prize patient'?

2 What happened to make Baker's temperature rise?

3 What do you learn about the problems facing surgeons on the Western Front?

Source F

Four photographs documenting the facial reconstruction of a soldier whose cheek was extensively wounded during the Battle of the Somme (July 1916).

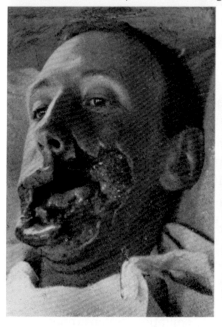
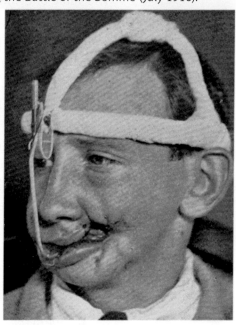
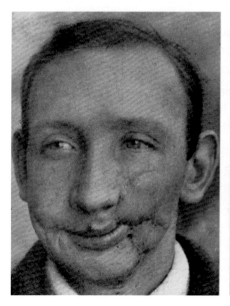
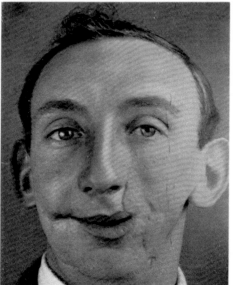

Source G

A photograph showing the work of Harold Gillies, 1916.

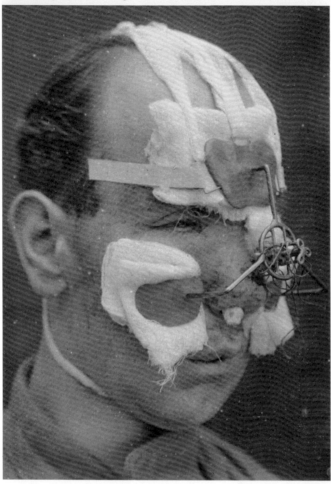

Source H

From *A Surgeon's Journal 1915–18*, by Harvey Cushing, published in 1936. This work is made up of extracts from the journal kept by American surgeon Cushing during the war. Here he is describing his first impressions of medical treatment on the Western Front soon after his arrival in France on 2 April 1915.

It is difficult to say just what are one's most vivid impressions: the amazing patience of the most seriously wounded, some of them hanging on for months; the dreadful deformities (not so much in the way of amputations, but broken jaws and twisted, scarred faces); the tedious healing of infected wounds with discharging sinuses, tubes, irrigation and repeated dressings. Painful fractures are simply abandoned to wait for wounds to heal, which they don't seem to do.

The intricate operations and recovery that were required in plastic surgery could not be carried out in France. Men who needed this surgery were returned to Britain. From August 1917, the key hospital providing this type of surgery was the Queen's Hospital in Sidcup, Kent. Gillies was involved in creating the design for the hospital so that it exactly matched his needs.

By the time of the end of the war, just over a year after the hospital opened, nearly 12,000 operations had been carried out.

THINKING HISTORICALLY ▶ **Evidence (3a)**

The value of evidence

Read Source H, then work through these tasks.

1 Write down at least two ways in which Cushing's memoir is useful for explaining injuries on the Western Front.

2 Compare your answers with a partner, then try to come up with at least one limitation of the source.

3 With your partner, decide how useful this source is for explaining injuries on the Western Front on a scale of 1 to 10 (10 being very useful).

4 What if the source was used to answer the question: 'How is Cushing's memoir useful for explaining the work done by surgeons and doctors on the Western Front?'

   a Write down any ways in which the source is useful for answering this new question.

   b Write down any limitations for answering the new question.

   c With your partner, decide how useful this source is for answering the question on a scale of 1 to 10.

   d Can you think of another enquiry for which this would be a useful source? Write it down and score the source on a scale of 1 to 10.

5 Compare your scores out of 10. How does the question being asked affect how useful a source is? Explain your answer.

6 Can you think of any other factors that might affect the usefulness of the source?

Activities

1 Make a list of the improvements in medical techniques that occurred on the Western Front.

2 Divide this list into those improvements that were linked to medical practice and those that involved other factors.

3 What are the other factors that contributed to medical improvements?

Summary

- Many new medical techniques and ideas were pioneered to meet the needs of those wounded on the Western Front.
- The Thomas splint was responsible for a dramatic decline in the number of deaths of men who received leg wounds.
- Mobile x-ray units enabled surgeons to see where shrapnel and bullets remained in the body. This reduced the number of deaths from infection by gas gangrene.
- The first use of stored blood in blood transfusions was at the Battle of Cambrai.
- Harvey Cushing developed new methods of brain surgery.
- Harold Gillies developed the effective use of plastic surgery for men who had suffered severe facial injuries.

Checkpoint

Strengthen

S1 List the different medical techniques used to treat the wounded on the Western Front.

S2 Explain the significance of the Blood Bank at Cambrai.

S3 What can you learn about plastic surgery from Sources G and H?

Challenge

C1 Look at the ways in which medical techniques improved. Which of these improvements do you think was the most important on the Western Front? Explain your answer to a partner. Do you agree with each other?

C2 How useful are Sources A and B as a study on treatment on the Western Front?

If you are not confident about any of these questions, form a group with other students, discuss the answers and then record your conclusions. Your teacher can give you some hints.

There are three questions in this section of the exam paper. This recap section is structured around the demands of the three questions.

- The **Two features quiz** is designed to help you prepare for the first question, which is a factual recall question about an aspect of this section of the course. However, this isn't the only time you'll need factual recall in the examination, so making sure you have a clear factual framework for the British sector of the Western Front is important. When you are answering questions about the sources, you need to use your knowledge of the period and interpret the sources in the context of what was happening at that time.

- The **This source is useful for** table helps you prepare for the second question in the exam, which gives you two sources and asks you how useful they would be for a particular enquiry.

- The **What is the question?** table helps you prepare for the second and third questions – in both of these questions, thinking about the enquiry is vital.

- Finally, the **All about the details** table helps you think about the types of source and how they can be used for new enquiries.

Two features quiz

For each topic below, list as many facts or features as you can. Aim to have at least two features for every topic.

1. The trench system
2. Stretcher bearers
3. Ambulances
4. Trench foot
5. Gas attacks
6. RAMC
7. FANY
8. Dressing stations
9. Casualty Clearing Stations
10. Base Hospitals
11. The underground hospital at Arras
12. The Thomas splint
13. Blood transfusions
14. The blood bank at Cambrai
15. Plastic surgery

This source is useful for

Sources	Enquiry	The Historical Context	One way in which the each source is useful
H (page 147) and D (page 150)	What were conditions like in the trenches?	Trench warfare on the Western Front lasted for most of the war and conditions in them varied…	Source B is useful because it shows what a trench looked like. Source D describes some of the problems during a battle…
H (page 172) and F (page 161)	What were the problems involved in caring for the wounded on the Western Front?		
C (page 159) and A (page 138)	What was the attitude of the soldiers to the medical treatment that they received?		

What is the question?

Source	Enquiry it would be useful for (and why)	Enquiry it would not be useful for (and why)
A (page 154)	How medical care in the frontline was carried out – the ways in which emergency first aid was used to keep men alive.	What happened to wounded men once they were moved further back in the chain of evacuation.
A (page 147)		
D (page 150)		
C (page 155)		
C (page 168)		

All about the details

Source	Detail	Question I would ask	Type of source I would use	How this might help answer my question
B (page 166)	'They seldom come to England without having been treated previously at a base abroad.'	To what extent were stretcher cases treated on the Western Front before being sent to England?	Medical records, and testimonies from those working on the Western Front.	Source B only has a narrow view of treatment on the Western Front. Muir worked in England, and so does not know exactly the types of treatment 'stretcher cases' were given on the Western Front.
G (page 151)				
A (page 138)				

Preparing for your GCSE Paper 1 exam

Paper 1 overview

Paper 1 is in two sections, which examine the historic environment and the thematic study. Together they count for 30% of your History assessment. The questions on the historic environment section of the 'Medicine though time' paper are in Section A and are worth 10% of your History assessment. Allow about one-third of the examination time for Section A, making sure you leave enough time for Section B. There are an extra four marks for the assessment of spelling, punctuation and grammar (SPaG) in the last question of Section B.

History Paper 1	Historic Environment and Thematic Depth Study			Time 1 hour 15 minutes
Section A	Historic Environment	Answer 3 questions	16 marks	25 minutes
Section B	Thematic study	Answer 3 questions	32 marks + 4 SPaG marks	50 minutes

Section A The historic environment: The British sector of the Western Front, 1914–18

You need to answer Question 1 and Question 2, which is in two parts.

1 Describe two features of... (4 marks)

You are given a few lines to write about each feature. Allow five minutes to write your answer. This question is only worth four marks and you should keep the answer brief and not try to add more information on extra lines.

2 (a) How useful are Sources A and B for an enquiry into... (8 marks)

You are given two sources to evaluate. They are in a separate sources booklet so you can keep them in front of you while you write your answer. Allow 15 minutes for this question, to give yourself time to read both sources carefully. Make sure your answer refers to both sources. You should **analyse** the sources.

- What useful information do they give? Only choose points that are directly relevant to the enquiry in the question.
- What can you infer? Work out what evidence they can provide that is not actually stated in the source.

You must also **evaluate** the source.

- Use contextual knowledge to evaluate the accuracy or completeness of the evidence.
- Use the provenance (the nature, origin and purpose of the source), to evaluate the strength of the evidence.

Make judgements about the usefulness of each source, giving clear reasons. These should be based on the importance of the content of the sources and should also take account of the provenance of the source.

Analyse
Information points
Inferences

+

Evaluate
Using knowledge
Using provenance

2 (b) Study Source... How could you follow up Source... to find out more about... ? (4 marks)

You are given a table to complete when you answer this question. It has four parts to it:

- the detail you would follow up
- the question you would ask
- the type of source you could use to find the information
- your explanation of how this information would help answer the question.

Allow five minutes to write your answer. You should keep your answer brief and not try to fill extra lines. The question is only worth four marks. Plan your answer so that all the parts link. Your answer will not be strong if you choose a detail to follow up, but then cannot think of a question or type of source that would help you follow it up.

Paper 1, Question 1

Describe **two** features of Casualty Clearing Stations.

(4 marks)

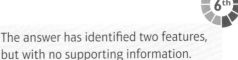

Exam tip

Keep your answer brief. Two points with some extra information about each feature is all you need.

Average answer

Casualty Clearing Stations were as close as possible to the frontline. The wounded were divided into three groups in the Casualty Clearing Stations.

The answer has identified two features, but with no supporting information.

Verdict

This is an average answer because two valid features are given, but there is no supporting information. Use the feedback to rewrite this answer, making as many improvements as you can.

Strong answer

Casualty Clearing Stations needed to be close enough to the frontline to be able to deal quickly with the wounded, but far enough away to have some protection from shelling.
A triage system was used to divide the wounded into groups in the clearing stations. Those who were not likely to survive would only be made comfortable, but not treated.

The answer has identified two features and describes them in more detail. The location of the Casualty Clearing Stations is described very clearly. The system of sorting patients is given its technical name and an example of one group is described.

Verdict

This is a strong answer because it gives two clear features of Casualty Clearing Stations and gives extra detail to make the descriptions more precise.

Sources for use with Section A

Source A

From Harvey Cushing's *A Surgeon's Journal 1915–18*, published in 1936. This work included extracts from the journal kept by Cushing, an American surgeon. Here he is describing the conditions under which he is working during the battle of Passchendaele on August 19 1917.

My prize patient, Baker, with the shrapnel ball removed from his brain, after doing well for three days suddenly shot up a temperature to 104 last night about midnight. I took him to the operating theatre, reopened the perfectly healed external wound, and found to my dismay a massive gas infection of the brain. I bribed two orderlies to stay up with him in the operating room, where he could have constant thorough irrigation over the brain and through the track of the missile [passing a warm saline solution along the path taken by the shrapnel to prevent infection]. No light except candles was permitted last night.

Source B

Photograph of a mobile x-ray unit taken in 1917.

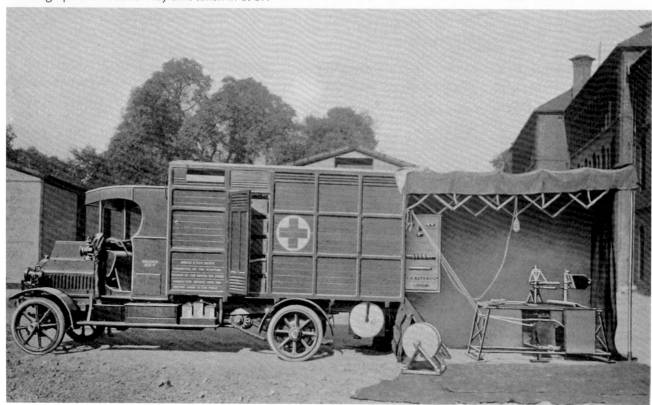

Paper 1, Question 2a

Study Sources A and B on page 178.
How useful are Sources A and B for an enquiry into the treatments that were available for wounded soldiers on the Western Front?
Explain your answer, using Sources A and B and your own knowledge of the historical context.   **(8 marks)**

Exam tip

Consider the strengths and weaknesses of the evidence. Your evaluation must link to the enquiry and use contextual knowledge. Your reasons (criteria) for judgement should be clear. Include points about:

- what information is relevant and what you can infer from the source
- how the provenance (the nature, origin and purpose) of each source affects its usefulness.

Average answer

Source A is useful because Cushing tells us that there were operating theatres where the wounded could be taken to be operated on at any time, even at night. There were staff available to keep watch on patients, although they had to be bribed to do this.

Source A is also useful because Cushing was a surgeon who carried out operations during the war and was at Passchendaele, although it is also not useful because this was published nearly 20 years after the end of the war. He is describing brain surgery and this was only one type of surgery. Other types of surgery were needed for other injuries, like leg and arm amputations.

Source B is useful because it is an actual photograph of a mobile x-ray machine that was used on the Western Front during the war to find shrapnel in the body. It is reliable because we know that these machines were carried around in vans and set up wherever they were needed. The photograph shows how the x-ray machine was linked to the van and the machine got its power from the van. It only shows one x-ray machine, so this makes it less useful.

Some useful information is taken from the source. The answer suggests an inference – 'operated on at any time', but does not really explain or develop this.

Comments are made about the author of the source, but they assume that the later publication date makes this unreliable. Additional knowledge shows an awareness of other types of operation, but is rather undeveloped.

These comments show that there is information that can be taken from the photograph. Knowledge is added to show that the photograph is reliable. It would be stronger with more developed evaluation.

Verdict

This is an average answer because:

- it has taken relevant information from both sources and shown some analysis by beginning to make an inference (so it is not a weak answer)
- it has added in some relevant contextual knowledge and used it for some evaluation of both the sources, but this is not sufficiently developed
- it does not explain criteria for judgement clearly enough to be a strong answer. The evaluation using the provenance of the sources should be more developed.

Use the feedback to rewrite this answer, making as many improvements as you can.

Paper 1, Question 2a

How useful are Sources A and B for an enquiry into the treatments that were available for wounded soldiers on the Western Front? **(8 marks)**

Strong answer

Source A is an account by Cushing of his wartime experiences as a brain surgeon. We can see that Cushing wanted patients to have the best possible treatment. He was prepared to 'bribe two orderlies' to keep watch on Baker. Cushing was extremely successful in treating brain injuries in 1917 when his patients had a survival rate of 71% (compared to the 50%, which was more normal for brain surgery), so it is likely that he is not exaggerating the care he gave to his patients. Although this account was published nearly 20 years after the war, it is still very useful because it was based on Cushing's journal. As an experienced surgeon, he probably kept the journal regularly and so this final work will record quite accurately what he was doing. He also probably remembered this patient very well because he refers to him as his 'prize patient'. Although this extract is only describing one surgeon and one patient's experiences in one type of surgery, it does point to some other information about treatment. The reference to gas gangrene ('massive gas infection') is important because we know that many men, even with quite minor injuries, suffered from this. If it was not treated in time by removal of tissue or use of antiseptics, the only way to save a man's life was amputation of the infected part of the body. This source also suggests problems with the conditions under which treatment took place. The operation took place at night, and the only light came from 'candles'.

Source B is useful because it shows a different way wounds were evaluated before treatment – x-rays. It is useful because it shows an example of a mobile x-ray machine, which was used on the Western Front, with the van that it was carried in. The machine is laid out under the tent at the back of the van, which is where a stretcher would be laid. You can see tubes connecting the x-ray machine to the van. This is because the machine was powered by the engine. The photo shows us what the van and the machine looked like, but we cannot tell from it how useful these machines actually were or how widely they were used. It does not tell us that there were only six of these machines in the British sector although there were also some static x-ray machines at the Base Hospitals, but it is useful to show that machines like the one in the photo were made available to some men on the frontline to improve chances of surviving.

Good analysis of the source linked to relevant knowledge. There is knowledge not just of different types of treatment that are available but also of the work done by Cushing himself and this own knowledge is used to support the comments on the provenance of the source.

Strengths and limitations of the source are shown and contextual knowledge is used in the evaluation, which also comments on the nature of the source.

Verdict

This is a strong answer because:
- it has analysed both sources, making inferences from them
- it has used contextual knowledge in the evaluation of both sources
- evaluation takes provenance into account and explains criteria clearly.

Paper 1, Question 2b

Study Source A (see page 178).
How could you follow up Source A to find out more about the treatments that were available for wounded soldiers on the Western Front?
In your answer, you must give the question you would ask and the type of source you could use.
Complete the table below.

(4 marks)

Average answer

Detail in Source A that I would follow up:
After doing well for three days a massive gas infection set in.
Question I would ask:
What other treatments could be used to deal with infections?

What type of source I could use:
Army medical records about treatments for infections.
How this might help answer my question:
It would describe the other types of treatment for infections.

The question is linked to the detail to be followed up.

The explanation of the type of source is restating the question, rather than a developed explanation.

Verdict

This is an average answer because the explanation of the question is not developed.
Use the feedback to rewrite this answer, making as many improvements as you can.

Strong answer

Detail in Source A that I would follow up:
After doing well for three days a massive gas infection set in.
Question I would ask:
How effective were the different types of treatments for dealing with infections like gas gangrene?

What type of source I could use:
Army medical records with statistical data on the survival rates of men who had different treatments for gas gangrene such as irrigation, debridement and amputation.
How this might help answer my question:
It would help to see if one of the treatments that was used on the Western Front was more effective than the others.

The answer has given a question linked directly to the issue identified.

The explanation is linked back to the question for follow-up and the type of source chosen.

Verdict

This is a strong answer because connections between the source details, the question and the source are securely linked.

Answers to Medicine Recap Questions

Chapter 1

1 To test someone's faith or punish them for sin
2 Galen and Hippocrates.
3 Blood, phlegm, black bile, yellow bile or choler
4 They had to become imbalanced
5 Answers could include the position of the stars and miasma
6 A spice-based mixture that could contain up to 70 ingredients, which was used as a cure to many diseases
7 *Regimen Sanitatis*
8 An alternative to a doctor or to mix remedies
9 1,100
10 One million

Chapter 2

1 Answers could include Jan Baptiste van Helmont, William Harvey and Robert Hooke
2 Thomas Sydenham refused to rely on medical books when diagnosing a patient's illness. Instead, he closely observed the symptoms and treating the disease causing them instead
3 The printing press
4 *Philosophical Transactions*
5 The science of looking for chemical cures
6 Syphilis had spread quickly in bath houses, making people scared to use them
7 300
8 Either a pest house, or nowhere. They were kept at home, quarantined for 28 days
9 William Harvey
10 Answers could include prayers or quarantine.

Chapter 3

1 Movements such as the Enlightenment made it fashionable to seek answers to questions about the world
2 Spontaneous generation
3 Pasteur's Germ Theory encouraged other scientists to look for alternatives to spontaneous generation
4 Microbes that caused tuberculosis and cholera
5 Treatments for everyday diseases, such as syphilis and tuberculosis, were not successfully developed until after 1900
6 Crimean War
7 Ether and chloroform
8 Answers could include providing clean water to stop the diseases that were spread in dirty water; disposing of sewage to prevent drinking and washing water from becoming polluted; and building public toilets to avoid pollution
9 1798
10 The Broad Street pump in Soho

Chapter 4

1 Franklin, Watson and Crick
2 2000
3 More powerful microscopes
4 1956 and 1968
5 Answers could include blood tests, x-rays, and progress in genetics
6 Hata, Salvarsan 606; Gerhard Domagk, Prontosil
7 Hospitals, General Practitioners (GPs) and dentists, (otherwise known as primary care), additional services, such as the ambulance service and health visitors and hospitals managed by regional hospital boards
8 Answers could include diphtheria and polio
9 Fleming, Florey and Chain
10 Surgery, transplants, radiotherapy, chemotherapy

Index